SIRTFOOD

DIET

THE COMPLETE GUIDE WITH
OVER 100 DELICIOUS AND
EASY RECIPES TO HELP YOU
EFFECTIVELY LOSE WEIGHT,
BURN FAT AND GET LEAN

By

Sam Gareth

Thanks for choosing this book. I wish you a good read and, if you like, leave a short review on Amazon.

Thank you

TABLE OF CONTENTS

INTRODUCTION

Fashionable brand-new diets appear to pop up regularly, and the Sirtfood Diet is among the most recent.

It has become a favorite of stars in Europe and is popular for allowing red wine and chocolate.

Its creators firmly insist that it's not a fad, however rather than "sirtfoods" are the secret to unlocking weight loss and avoiding disease.

Nevertheless, health specialists caution that this diet might not measure up to the hype and might even be a bad concept.

A diet that does not include fasting 2 days a week and yet declares to bring numerous of the exact the same advantages as the 5:2 diet plan? A diet plan where typical weight loss is 7lb in the very first 7 days? I felt I had to inspect the

Sirtfood Diet out

So I chose the only reasonable thing to do for a food blog writer like me was to give it a completely excellent trial and see if the diet is as great as it declares to be ...(and I guarantee I wasn't encouraged by the coffee, red wine, and chocolate ... truthful!

Sirtfoods are a just recently found group of nutrient abundant foods which appear to be able to 'trigger' the body's skinny genes (likewise called sirtuins), in much the same way as fasting diets do, with the very same range of benefits, but without the common drawbacks of fasting diet plans, such as cravings, irritation and muscle loss.

Is it good to be real? Here's everything you require to understand about the Sirtfood Diet, from the science behind it to fresh recipe ideas to try Adele's weight-loss has been all anybody can speak about just recently after pictures emerged of the vocalist holidaying on a beach in Anguilla three stone lighter.

How did she accomplish it? Apparently by taking up the Sirtfood Diet-- well-known for actively motivating those following it to have red wine and chocolate.

The Sirtfood diet has ended up being as huge recently as the Cabbage Soup diet plan, the 5.2 Diet and Dukan diet, popular not just with Adele, however, stars like Lorraine Pascale and Jodie Kidd too. But is it yet another diet that promises excessive, or can following a sirtfood eating plan help you lose weight and feel better?

We've separated reality from fiction to bring you everything you require to understand about the Sirtfood Diet

WHAT IS A SIRTFOOD?

What sounds like a treat lifted directly from a sci-fi movie, a 'sirtfood' is a food high in sirtuin activators. Sirtuins are a type of protein that secures the cells in our bodies from dying or becoming irritated through a health problem, though research study has also shown they can assist manage your metabolic process, increase muscle and burn fat-- hence the new 'wonder food' tag.

Sirtfoods are all easily offered and accessible foods and some of the top Sirtfoods include kale, rocket, parsley, red onions, strawberries, walnuts, additional virgin olive oil, cocoa, curry spices, green tea and coffee (yes, coffee!). In contrast to previous popularised diet plans where the focus is on cutting out foods, with Sirtfoods the advantages are reaped through consuming.

Together with fat-burning, Sirtfoods also have the unique ability to naturally satiate appetite and boost muscle function making them the best option to attaining a healthy weight. And their health-enhancing effects are so powerful that research studies reveal them to be more effective than prescription drugs in avoiding chronic illness, with benefits in diabetes, cardiovascular disease, and Alzheimer's to call simply a couple of. It's no marvel that it is well developed that the cultures eating the most Sirtfoods have been the cleanest and healthiest in the world.

Over the past couple of years, fasting diets have been the biggest craze, especially ones like the 5:2 diet, which was the-diet-to-do in 2015.

The Sirtfood plan is expected to stimulate the weight loss results of a fasting diet plan-- but without jeopardizing health, fitness, muscle mass or food satisfaction, thanks to new research study into this food group. Simply in case 500-calorie Mondays (AKA starving-all-day Mondays) weren't truly working out for you.

Although being an effective weight loss routine, the authors are keen to tension that it isn't merely a diet strategy, however a wellbeing and fitness routine.

" It does not require calorie restriction, nor does it require grueling exercise regimes (although obviously, remaining generally active is an excellent thing. It's neither costly nor lengthy, and all the foods we recommend are commonly readily available."

And yes, because list includes dark chocolate (cocoa) and red wine - rejoice!

It's the buzz diet of 2016, and already a favorite amongst stars, with everyone from Jodie Kidd to Lorraine Pascal liking it.

Lorraine called it "a non-faddy diet plan that uses incredible health benefits and weight-loss."

Jodie said: "Since following it, I feel unstoppable."

But how exactly do these foods work to attain such extreme results?

HOW THE SIRTFOOD DIET WORKS

Sirtfoods work by activating so-called "slim gene" paths in the body, the same genes that are activated when we work out or quick.

This helps the body to burn fat in a manner that mimics calories limitation, but without the nutrition loss or other drawbacks.

A typical loss of 7 pounds of weight in 7 days was reported by the sample of individuals testing the diet, together with increased muscle mass and reports of feeling satisfied and complete with food intake.

The book describes that the Sirtfoods operate in the following method:

" Sirtfoods act as master regulators of our whole metabolism, most notably having impacts on fat loss while concurrently increasing muscle and boosting cellular physical fitness."

Throughout their research, Goggins and Matten discovered that many of the foods that fall under the Stirfood category are already frequently connected with the healthiest diets worldwide - as the common Mediterranean diet.

There are 2 phases to the plan listed in the book, with the very first being the more intense '7ibs-in-7-days' part, and the 2nd looking more into the maintenance side of things.

What can you eat on the Sirtfood Diet?

As highlighted in The Official Sirtfood Diet, the diet plan program is based on a meal plan that is curated to be full of sirtfoods, but cut in overall calorie counts. The book's meal strategy is quite regimented: For the first 3 days, dieters are expected to consume simply 1,000 calories each day that consists of a single meal and two green juices.

The bulk of the program asks dieters to develop meals that are high in sirtfoods ... and very little else. A few of the staples that the diet highlight consist of several fruit and vegetable products, including kale, strawberries, onions, parsley, arugula, blueberries, and capers. Some grains, like buckwheat, and walnuts are praised, as are spices like turmeric. Interestingly, drinks like coffee, matcha green tea, and red white wine are motivated-- as is a heavy reliance on 85% dark chocolate.

Is the Sirtfood Diet healthy for you?

You're not alone-- lots of health specialists criticize the Sirtfood Diet for being highly limiting if the diet plan's list of well-known ingredients seems a bit doing not have. Since it's tight calorie constraints, Beckerman states she has never recommended the Sirtfood Diet to any of her customers. "While I praise the Sirtfood Diet for promoting the usage of genuine active ingredients, I denounce it for its promo of calorie limitation and unhealthy consuming rules." Like numerous other diets that eliminate food groups from regular consumption, Beckerman says the Sirtfood Diet may certainly lead to "disordered eating" as it also blends elements from periodic fasting strategies into the mix.

McKenzie Caldwell, MPH, RDN, who specializes in ladies' nutrition and pregnancy dietary health in specific, states that the calorie counts associated with the diet plan are without a doubt it's the worst quality. "1,000 calories daily is just proper for a child between the ages of 2 and 4," she says, mentioning present dietary guidelines distributed by the Mayo Clinic. "Not only is this insufficient energy to support an adult body, but it also is not possible to suit all the macro- and micronutrient adult requirements because of the amount of food ... The diet plan may cause weight-loss in the short-term merely since of its calorie constraint."

Most significantly, nevertheless, both nutrition specialists agree that there is little to no clinical proof to support this diet plan being healthy for sustained weight-loss. "There is absolutely no proof to back up any claims that the Sirtfood Diet has a beneficial impact on healthy weight loss," Beckerman says. "The developers of the diet claim to have put participants at their gym on the diet, however, this anecdotal supposed study has not been released nor verified by true scientists or scientists."

This diet plan is based on a research study on sirtuins (SIRTs), a group of seven proteins found in the body that has been revealed to control a variety of functions, consisting of swelling, metabolic process, and life expectancy (1Trusted Source).

Specific natural plant substances may have the ability to increase the level of these proteins in the body, and foods including them have been called "sirtfoods".

The list of the "top 20 sirtfoods" offered by the Sirtfood Diet includes:

Kale.

Red white wine.

Strawberries.

Onions.

Soy.

Parsley.

Bonus virgin olive oil.

Dark chocolate (85% cocoa).

Matcha green tea.

Buckwheat.

Turmeric.

Walnuts.

Arugula (rocket).

Bird's eye chili.

Lovage.

Medjool dates.

Red chicory.

Blueberries.

Capers.

Coffee.

The diet plan combines sirtfoods and calorie restriction, both of which may activate the body to produce greater levels of sirtuins.

This sirtfood diet book includes meal plans and dishes to follow, however, there are plenty of other Sirtfood Diet recipe books readily available.

The diet plan's creators claim that following the Sirtfood Diet will cause rapid weight loss, all while keeping muscle mass and securing you from persistent illness.

As soon as you have completed the diet plan, you are motivated to continue including sirtfoods and the diet plan's signature green juice into your regular diet plan.

The Sirtfood Diet is based upon a research

study on sirtuins, a group of proteins that manage numerous functions in the body. Specific foods called sirtfoods might cause the body to produce more of these proteins.

IS IT EFFECTIVE?

The authors of the Sirtfood Diet make bold claims, including that the diet can super-charge weight-loss, switch on your "slim gene" and avoid illness.

The issue exists isn't much proof to back them.

Far, there's no convincing proof that the Sirtfood Diet has a more beneficial impact on weight loss than any other calorie-restricted diet.

And although numerous of these foods have healthful homes, there have not been any long-lasting human research studies to determine whether eating a diet rich in sirtfoods has any concrete health benefits.

Nonetheless, this sirtfood diet plan book reports the outcomes of a pilot study conducted by the authors and involving 39 individuals from their gym. Nevertheless, the results of this study appear not to have been published anywhere else.

For one week, the individuals followed the diet and worked out daily. At the end of the week, participants lost approximately 7 pounds (3.2 kg) and kept or perhaps gained muscle mass.

Yet these outcomes are hardly surprising. Restricting your calorie intake to 1,000 calories and working out at the very same time will almost always trigger weight reduction.

Regardless, this type of quick weight-loss is neither lasting nor genuine, and this study did not follow participants after the very first week to see if they got any of the weight back, which is normally the case.

When your body is energy-deprived, it utilizes up its emergency energy stores, or glycogen, in addition to burning fat and muscle.

Each particle of glycogen needs 3-- 4 particles of water to be kept. When your body uses up glycogen, it gets rid of this water also. It's known as "water weight."

In the first week of extreme calorie constraint, just about one-third of the weight-loss comes from fat, while the other two-thirds comes from water, muscle, and glycogen

As quickly as your calorie intake boosts, your body renews its glycogen shops, and the weight comes right back.

This type of calorie limitation can likewise cause your body to decrease its metabolic rate, triggering you require even fewer calories per day for energy than before

It is most likely that this diet plan may assist you to lose a couple of pounds in the beginning, but it will likely come back as quickly as the diet plan is over.

As far as avoiding illness, 3 weeks is probably not long enough to have any measurable long-lasting effect.

On the another hand, adding sirtfoods to your regular diet over the long-term might well be a good idea. In that case, you may as well avoid the diet and begin doing that now.

This diet may assist you to drop weight since it is low in calories, but the weight is most likely to return when the diet plan ends. The diet plan is too short to have a long-term impact on your health.

HOW TO FOLLOW THE SIRTFOOD DIET

The Sirtfood Diet has two stages that last overall of three weeks. After that, you can continue "sirtifying" your diet by including as numerous sirtfoods as possible in your meals.

The particular dishes for these two stages are discovered in This sirtfood diet plan book, which was composed of the diet plan's creators. You'll need to buy it to follow the diet.

The meals have lots of sirtfoods, however, do consist of other active ingredients besides simply the "top 20 sirtfoods."

Most of the sirtfoods and ingredients are simple to discover.

Nevertheless, 3 of the signature ingredients needed for these 2 stages-- matcha green tea powder, lovage, and buckwheat-- might be costly or difficult to discover.

A big part of the diet is its green juice, which you'll need to make yourself in between one and 3 times daily. You will require a juicer (a blender will not work) and a cooking area scale, as the components are listed by weight. The recipe is listed below:

Sirtfood Green Juice

75 grams (2.5 oz) kale

30 grams (1 oz) arugula (rocket).

5 grams parsley.

2 celery sticks.

1 cm (0.5 in) ginger.

half a green apple.

half a lemon.

half a teaspoon matcha green tea.

Juice all active ingredients except for the green tea powder and lemon together, and put them into a glass. Juice the lemon by hand, then stir both the lemon juice and green tea powder into your juice.

Phase One.

The first stage lasts seven days and involves calorie limitation and lots of green juice. It is meant to jump-start your weight reduction and declared to help you lose 7 pounds (3.2 kg) in seven days.

Throughout the very first three days of phase one, calorie consumption is restricted to 1,000 calories. You consume 3 green juices per day plus one meal. Every day you can pick from dishes in the book, which all involve sirtfoods as the main part of the meal.

Meal examples include miso-glazed tofu, the sirtfood omelet, or a shrimp stir-fry with buckwheat noodles.

On days 4-- 7 of stage one, calorie consumption is increased to 1,500. This consists of two green juices per day and two more sirtfood-rich meals, which you can select from the book.

Stage Two.

Stage two lasts for two weeks. Throughout this "maintenance" stage, you need to continue to steadily drop weight.

There is no specific calorie limitation for this phase. Rather, you consume three meals loaded with sirtfoods and one green juice per day. Again, the meals are picked from dishes offered in the book.

After the Diet.

You may repeat these two stages as often as

preferred for more weight loss.

Nevertheless, you are motivated to continue "sirtifying" your diet plan after completing these phases by including sirtfoods frequently into your meals.

There are a variety of Sirtfood Diet books that have plenty of recipes abundant in sirtfoods. You can also consist of sirtfoods in your diet as a treat or in dishes you already utilize.

Also, you are encouraged to continue drinking green juice every day.

In this method, the Sirtfood Diet becomes more of a way of life change than a one-time diet plan.

The Sirtfood Diet consists of 2 phases. Stage one lasts 7 days and combines calorie limitation and green juices. Phase 2 lasts two weeks and includes 3 meals and one juice.

THE SIRTFOOD MEAL PLAN STEPS AND 3 WEEKS PLAN SAMPLE (PERSONAL EXPERIENCE)

> ## SIRTFOOD DIET WEEK 1 SAMPLE
>
> - ### DAY 1/ MONDAY (3 JUICES, 1 MEAL).

Well, having got to grips with my brand-new juicer and done a bit of shopping to begin myself off, I was ready and getting ready to go. The first 3 days of the Sirtfood Diet involve 3 green juices and only 1 meal, so I was gotten ready for it to be difficult, but actually, I was happily amazed. The juices were drinkable and bizarrely I didn't feel starving throughout the day till about 5 pm (which was only an hour before supper, so bearable).

Sirtfood Diet Green Juice Recipe.

Supper was this tasty King Prawn Stir Fry with

Buckwheat Noodles ...

King Prawn Stir Fry with Buckwheat Noodles.

The genuine highlight of the day was the two squares of Lindt 85% chocolate I was enabled after supper. I waited until my kids remained in bed and I had finished work for the day before I allowed myself this reward and it was fabulous but did seem rather naughty!

Lindt 85% Dark Chocolate for the Sirtfood Diet.

I spaced the juices out so I had one at 7.30 am (our usual breakfast time), one at 11 am, one at 2.30 pm and after that dinner at 6 pm and the chocolate at about 9 pm. Before heading off to bed I made up my 3 juices for the next day.

What is the very best juicer for The Sirtfood Diet?

- DAY 2/ TUESDAY (3 JUICES, 1 MEAL).

The juice, which I had been quite delighted drinking on Monday, tasted disgusting-- so much so that it made me gag! I have a few theories: maybe making it up the night before meant the juices were less fresh, perhaps the kale I used in batch 2 of the juices was a bit previous its finest, maybe my body had all of a sudden changed its mind and rejected the juice? I had a couple of sips and then the rest of juice 3 went down the sink.

Sirtfood Diet Green Juice Recipe.

On the plus side, I still didn't feel starving at all. All-day! Not even at 5 pm, like the day previously. And the dinner I picked: Kale and Red Onion Dhal with Buckwheat were delicious. Each day there are 2 choices for supper: a meat/fish one and a veggie/vegan one.

I choose to match a bit and blend depending on what the options were. The dhal sounded so good, I just needed to try it and I was not dissatisfied.

Kale and Red Onion Dhal from the Sirtfood Diet.

And naturally, there was that terrific decadent treat of two squares of Lindt 85%. I decided after my green juice catastrophe that I would not make I energize the night in the past, but instead make them up fresh each time on Wednesday. Also, Tesco Man showed up with a fresh batch of kale so the old manky kale went in the bin.

- DAY 3/ WEDNESDAY (3 JUICES, 1 MEAL).

I made a couple of changes to the juice on Wednesday. I a little up the apple-- an entire one, not half according to the recipe. And I a little reduced the celery-- the primary smell that was making me gag. I lowered the celery down from 2 to 1 stick. Otherwise I just made up the juice the like Monday and Tuesday ... and it was fine! I'm not going to lie to you, it's not the most delicious thing I've ever drunk in my life, but it is perfectly drinkable (unlike Tuesday's bad batch which certainly was not!).

Sirtfood Green Juice as a Salad.

Nevertheless, a thought had been worrying in my brain because the start of the diet ... the Sirtfood green juice active ingredients all sounded like rather fab ingredients for a salad ... would it work? Well, I figured it deserved a shot! Rather than juice 2, I used the ingredients to make an easy salad. I made a dressing out of the lemon juice and ginger and a tiny bit of additional virgin olive oil. I rubbed it into the kale and then included the rocket, celery, apple, and parsley, plus a couple of walnuts. Both walnuts and extra virgin olive oil are Sirtfoods, so I didn't feel too naughty adding them ... and yes it did make a lovely salad (recipe below, if you expensive it). The salad was massive-- I could not complete it all and taste beautiful. Certainly, one to have once again and much better than the juice!!

Wednesday's supper was another victory: Aromatic Chicken with Kale, Buckwheat, and Salsa. It was extremely easy and delicious to do. And the salsa ... I could have consumed a whole bucket of that-- soo excellent! My only complaint would be that it used every pot and pan in your home (OKAY I exaggerate. It utilized 5. However that is way more than I would typically use-- I am a 1 pot kind of a girl, often 2 but NEVER 5, unless it's like Christmas or something and even then ... have you saw my Christmas Turkey Traybake Recipe?). I think whoever writes the Sirtfood dishes should have somebody who does his cleaning up for him. (Quick check of the book reveals it's a chef called Mark McCulloch ... so he probably does have a whole army of underlings to clean up for him!).

Aromatic Chicken Breast with Kale and Red Onions and a Tomato and Chilli Salsa from the Sirtfood Diet.

And after that, there was the chocolate once again. You have to picture me at about 9 pm, on the couch, reading a book, eating chocolate, and drinking camomile tea. I'm so very delighted. It's an extremely, extremely good way to end the day!

- DAY 4/ THURSDAY (2 JUICES, 2 MEALS).

So on Day 4 all of its modifications and you are enabled 2 proper meals and 2 green juices. This offered me a little bit of a predicament as to when to have the first meal, which on Thursday was the Sirt Muesli-- more of a breakfast thing really, but I wished to spread out the meals out a bit so I chose to have the muesli at 11 am and the juices at 7.30 am and 2.30 pm.

Sirt Muesli from the Sirtfood Diet.

As before, I made the juice up fresh to my a little adapted dish and it was great. Making the juice sounds a bit of a faff, however, truly it isn't. It takes all of 10 minutes to drink the juice and make and do the washing up when you get utilized to it. That's quicker than my typical breakfast (of 2 shredded wheat and a glass of orange juice) takes to consume (I'm a slow eater, OK!). I do believe one of the important things that made the green juice so manageable was my fab Juicer. It is really simple to wash and utilize up. I really love it and will certainly be making more juices once I've finished the Sirtfood Diet (though possibly I'll take a break from ones including kale and celery for a while!).

The Sirt Muesli was FAB and one of the outright highlights of Week 1 (the other most certainly being Saturday's dinner! It's really quick to put together. You can make loads of it in one go.

For supper, I went with the vegan choice of Tuscan Bean Stew. (There is a salmon option, if you choose, which likewise sounds excellent.) The stew was extremely good, however, it was the third meal in a row served with buckwheat and it would have been great if it had been served with something else as I was getting a bit fed up with buckwheat by this point. Buckwheat is great but not every day. Ditto kale and celery for that matter. I know the Sirtfood Diet attempts to cram in as much of the leading 20 Sirtfoods as possible into each meal however it does produce a bit excessive sameyness. I do like kale/celery/buckwheat etc. But for breakfast lunch and dinner every day for a week-- not so much!

Tuscan Bean Stew from the Sirtfood Diet.

Now here's the important things. After Wednesday, there is no more mention of the Chocolate, which I reckon was a typo! So (extremely naughtily) I decided to continue with the Lindt 85%. Well ... it is a Sirtfood after all!

- DAY 5/ FRIDAY (2 JUICES, 2 MEALS).

Friday started, as all my other days, with a green juice, however, then it was school sports day and picnic, which had me in a bit of a predicament about how to do things. In the end, I chose to do the juices at home and take Meal 1-- a remarkably portable Strawberry Buckwheat Tabbouleh to the picnic.

Strawberry Buckwheat Tabbouleh from the Sirtfood Diet.

Strawberry Buckwheat Tabbouleh as a packed lunch from the Sirtfood Diet.

Supper was Miso Marinated Baked Cod and again, scrumptious but with yet more kale and buckwheat, a wee bit samey. It was starting to drive me a bit bonkers! And my bad kids. They were a bit cross about having to eat buckwheat once again. Especially as Friday night is generally pizza night ... oops!

Miso Marinated Baked Cod from the Sirtfood Diet.

And yes ... there was more chocolate. I'm sorry. I couldn't help myself!

- DAY 6/ SATURDAY (2 JUICES, 2 MEALS).

Today the kids and my husband were home, so

I had juice for breakfast and then the Sirtfood meals for lunch and supper. Lunch was the Sirtfood Super Salad, a delicious mix of rocket, chicory, avocado, walnuts, capers, and a whole host of other Sirtfoods.

Sirtfood Super Salad.

The real highlight of the day was dinner: Chargrilled Beef with Red Wine Gravy and Herby Roast Potatoes. That red white wine gravy was simply remarkable-- I'll certainly be making that again.

Chargrilled Beef with Red Wine Jus from the Sirtfood Diet.

Despite the diet being hailed as the red wine and chocolate diet plan, red white wine is strictly off-limits in Week 1 (thereafter you can have 2-3 glasses per week if you want). The fact there was red wine in the sauce did assistance. In my world, an excellent steak requires a good red wine!

- DAY 7/ SUNDAY (2 JUICES, 2 MEALS).

Sunday was a hectic day with lots going on in the morning and I knew lunch would be late. The thought of surviving till 2 pm on juice alone didn't appeal, so I cheated somewhat and had a bowl of that delicious Sirt Muesli rather. Oh my, that stuff is soo good!

Lunch was a wonderful Sirtfood Omelet with Bacon. Officially you are supposed to put the bacon IN the omelet however I had mine on the side instead. I simply had this (well, OK I might have had 3 slices of bacon ... however I had had an extremely busy early morning) and my kids and hubby had beans and toast.

Provided my children are not huge fans of red onions or tomatoes, I made a 'regular' salad for them and served it up with some crusty white bread for them and my husband, but I just ate the chicken and the red onion salad. I somewhat adjusted the salad by adding in some capers and utilizing lemon juice rather than red wine vinegar.

SIRTFOOD DIET WEEK 1: REFLECTIONS AND SUGGESTIONS

TOO MUCH FOOD/ PORTION SIZES/ RANDOM MEASUREMENTS

Most likely my greatest gripe with the Sirtfood Diet is the portion sizes are enormous, which appears to beat the object of a diet. I would much rather have two smaller meals in the day than one enormous one that I can't end up and often it's not the portions that appear supersized however the proportions-- like absurd amounts of kale with the steak or 2 boxes of cherry tomatoes in the salsa (if you make it for 4 that is). If you are going to do the Sirtfood Diet, I strongly advise you to use your sound judgment and do the amount that appears sensible to you, if the book suggests excessive food.

And actually, the authors do state in their second book that if you feel complete you need to stop eating and not force yourself to finish a part which is too big.

LACK OF VARIETY

I got completely fed up with kale, celery, and buckwheat in week 1. I like all 3, however by the end of Week 1, I sort of didn't any more! You can absolutely have too much of a great thing!! It would be good if there was a bit more range in the meal plan. I acknowledge to a particular extent, it was my fault changing in between the meat and vegan options. If you plan to match and mix, I do recommend you are cautious to prevent excessive sameyness. I will be more cautious next week.

WEIGHT REDUCTION AND OTHER BENEFITS

I lost 5lb in the very first 3 days !! And given how much I was consuming, I'm not sure it is possible that was from fluid loss. The unique thing about this diet plan is that it is supposed to help you get muscle as well as lose weight. I do not have expensive scales that tell me such things so, I can't comment on that, but in the book, they say typically individuals put on a little weight in muscle, as well as losing weight in fat, so it is entirely possible that I have put on muscle and lost even more fat.

But for me, the diet plan was a lot more than about reducing weight. I was intrigued to see if I might benefit from any of the other claims ... and the answer is likewise yes! I feel healthier, I've been sleeping much better, I feel more favorable and energetic, more alert (and no it's not since of the coffee-- I've intoxicated no more coffee than normal and most days less) and bizarrely I've also felt less starving than normal! I have also been consuming more water and I understand now that typically when I feel starving I'm probably, in fact, thirsty ... or simply tired!

> **SIRTFOOD DIET WEEK 2 SAMPLE**
   - DAY 8 MONDAY

It was so good to be back on 3 meals a day!! The juice part of the diet did its thing and helped me lose 6lb, and now comes the much more enjoyable part of the diet: the 'upkeep' phase! This part of the diet plan is a lot more of a healthy eating plan than a 'diet plan' per se. You are permitted 3 healthy Sirtfood meals a day plus 1 or 2 little treats. Drinks-wise you are still limited to green tea, coffee, black tea, and water, however, you are now allowed to have 2-3 glasses of red wine per week.

Today started with a Sirtfood Smoothie, which was okay, but not as great as the Sirtfood Muesli and it was a bit of a disappointment that after 7 days of rests breakfast, the first breakfast you are allowed remains in liquid form!

Lunch was far more interesting: I had another Chicken Sirtfood Super salad, which was just as nice as it was on Saturday. I had currently baked an additional chicken breast at Sunday supper time so this salad took simple minutes to throw together.

Dinner required to be flexible as my hubby was returning late, so I chose the veggie choice of Tuscan Bean Stew again, which was simple to make and tasted fantastic.

I generally stuck to the plan but switched in a couple of meals from The Sirtfood Diet Recipe Book. I was impressed at just how household-friendly The Sirtfood Diet Recipe Book is.

And yes, I did keep up my little Lindt 85% chocolate habit-- pretty much all week!

- DAY 9 TUESDAY

Breakfast was the terrific Sirtfood Muesli once again, which was as good as constantly. This is a fab way to begin the day and fills me up remarkably. I do not feel hungry once again up until lunch break.

Tuesday was the day of my daughter's school journey and I was going along as one of the moms and dad helpers, so I required to have something at lunch break that would work well as a jam-packed lunch. The lunch set up for Tuesday was wholemeal pittas. Perfect for a jam-packed lunch. I do however have a strong hostility to soggy sandwiches, so instead of making my pittas up in the morning, I loaded everything I would need for them and made them up at lunchtime, much to the amusement of my child's classmates!

After a busy day, our night meal was mercifully basic to toss together-- a scrumptious butternut squash and date tagine. I was a little concerned that with the butternut squash and the dates it would be too sweet, but in fact, it was ok and the sweet taste worked so well with the cinnamon. I would like to attempt this tagine again however with lamb in it too, as I can picture the cinnamon and dates would go so extremely well with lamb. (Edit: I did eventually remake this tagine with lamb and it was amazing!!

The tagine was served with yet more buckwheat, but, by this point, I was really beginning to get a taste for the buckwheat! I believe it's a little bit of an acquired taste and now I'm accustomed to it, I'm rather enjoying it. Even the kids didn't grumble this time!

- DAY 10 WEDNESDAY

For breakfast, I had Greek yogurt with mixed berries, chocolate, and walnuts-- a rather decadent treat for breakfast-- and much nicer than Monday's smoothie. (And way better than the green juices!). I added a couple of coconut flakes for additional scrumptiousness.

Sirtfood Breakfast of Yoghurt, Berries, Walnuts, Coconut Flakes and Cacao Nibs

Lunch was supposed to be the Sirtfood Supersalad once again, but still having some components left over from yesterday, I decided to have pittas once again. I think one way this diet plan could be enhanced is by recognizing that you might have some leftover components from the previous day and reusing them the next day.

The kids and I had a fun time making these scrumptious Sirtfood Bites after school. They are made from a mix of dates, cacao, walnuts, and turmeric, and taste amazing! You are supposed to have 1 to 2 a day. By the end of Wednesday, there were none left in our house-- I think the kids liked them then! Oh well, far much better for them than Haribo!!

I did manage to handle snaffle a couple. On Wednesday I usually choose a run with my jogging group so several Sirtfood Bites were simply ideal for giving me the energy for a 4.5-mile run ... Ok, so it was 4 Sirtfood Bites that I consumed. I figured I would burn them all off on my run, no?

Wednesday's dinner was a tasty chili con carne, which was simply best for a day when we were all eating at different times. I made the chili for the kids and then reheated it for my spouse and I later. The kids had it with white rice and spouse and I had ours with buckwheat. The chili was a relatively standard dish, however with a lot of sirtfoods from chili, red white wine, turmeric, and cocoa. It tasted magnificent, though not quite as nice as my Slow Cooked Chilli Beef. I believe I may attempt adding some cocoa, turmeric and red white wine into my Chilli Beef next time I make it, to up the Sirtfood material!

- DAY 11 THURSDAY

Thursday's breakfast was expected to be spiced scrambled eggs, but the idea of cooking and eating scrambled eggs at 7.30 on a busy school early morning just did not appeal, so I made the wonderful sirtfood muesli rather. To shake things up a little, I included a couple of blueberries and raspberries into the mix also.

Lunch was expected to be the strawberry buckwheat tabbouleh again, however, I chose I rather fancied having a go at something else, so rather I made this rather amazing potato salad to go with rainbow trout and watercress, a dish from The Sirtfood Recipe Book. I also added in a handful of rocket for additional Sirtfood goodness. Include a prepared fillet of smoked trout and a handful of watercress and you are great to go.

I was feeling a little peckish at about 4 pm and sadly we had polished off all the Sirtfood Bites the day previously. I didn't have time to make any more, so instead, I had a handful of walnuts and a date. I figured because they were both Sirtfoods and components in the Sirtfood Bites, they would make a good alternative. It would be nice to have a few suggestions for simple and quick treats in the books. The Sirtfood Diet Recipe Book does have several treat recipes, but no ideas for simple and quick snacks you do not need to make.

Chicken and Kale Curry with Bombay Potatoes from The Sirtfood Diet

Supper was one I had been anticipating considering that I initially began the diet plan: Chicken and Kale Curry with Bombay Potatoes. I a little adapted the dish, utilizing chicken thighs rather of breast fillets, but otherwise kept whatever broadly the same. It was a great adequate curry, however by no methods my preferred meal of the week and the Bombay potatoes were a bit uninteresting-- more like yellow roast potatoes than Bombay potatoes!

- DAY 12 FRIDAY

I did feel I might have overindulged on Thursday-- I ate quantities of both meals that were a little larger than I need to have, in addition to having that extra snack and low and witness when I weighed myself on Friday early morning I had put on a pound. Nevertheless, regardless of placing on a pound, I have still been gaining the benefits of a very healthy diet. I am still feeling quite 'bright-eyed and bushy-tailed' and continue to sleep incredibly well. My stomach is likewise flatter than it's remained in years!

Friday's breakfast was a re-run of Wednesdays, with Greek Yogurt, fresh fruit, cacao nibs, walnuts, and coconut flakes. Tasty and quickly kept me going until lunch. I need to have had the Sirtfood Smoothie, but I chose the yogurt and fruit choice would be much nicer-- and it was!

Sirtfood Breakfast of Yoghurt, Berries, Walnuts, Coconut Flakes and Cacao Nibs

For lunch, I decided to have the Sirtfood Super Salad, instead of the Waldorf Salad on the plan. I am enjoying the fact you can match and blend and switch in different things, depending upon what you expensive. This time I picked to have some leftover feta cheese rather of chicken in my salad. Although not an 'official' alternative, I had some left over from Wednesday's pittas and I knew it would go brilliantly with the other components, particularly the rocket, avocado, and walnuts-- and it did! I will be having this variation rather. I chose it for the chicken alternative.

I did attempt to keep the journal as complimentary as possible for the 3 weeks of the Sirtfood Diet, but it was difficult to discover 3 weeks with absolutely nothing organized and we had had this Friday's earmarked as a 'date night' for months. I expect I could have canceled it, however, my hubby and I have date nights so infrequently that, well, I didn't wish to! We decided to go ahead and go out to a restaurant as we had initially planned.

Nevertheless, this did offer me a little bit of a problem, Sirtfood-wise. There are absolutely no guidelines for what to do at a dining establishment in the book. Certainly, I could not phone the dining establishment and ask to make Buckwheat Pasta with Smoked Salmon, Chili, and Rocket, according to the plan! I decided to just go for little parts and just one glass of wine. We went to a lovely Thai dining establishment-- which was excellent as I understood I would get at least a few Sirtfoods, such as chili, shallots, herbs, nuts, and spices, as well as that very important glass of red wine. I also had a coffee afterward instead of pudding. And I can tell you, after 12 days of abstinence, that glass of red wine tasted great indeed!

- DAY 13 SATURDAY

I have been looking at my buckwheat flakes and questioning if they might make an excellent porridge all week, so chosen Saturday would be an excellent day to offer it a go. And shaved 5 minutes off my previous PB!!

Lunch was supposed to be Tofu and Shitake

Mushroom soup, which sounded nice to me, but couldn't envision else in my family would be particularly happy with it, so I swapped switched another recipe from The Sirtfood Diet Recipe

Book of Grilled Sausages with Herby Scrambled eggs. I slightly adjusted the recipe by including in some turmeric and chili to the scrambled eggs to make them additional Sirtfoodie!! My kids were not convinced and declined to try the eggs, rather plumping for toast and baked beans to go with their sausages.

Saturday night was even more difficult to handle than Friday night. We had been welcomed round to a friend's home for a murder secret party ... Where the menu was a seafood plate, followed by venison and mashed potato and after that a choice of desserts: pavlova or banoffee pie. All completely delicious, but barely a Sirtfood insight. Now clearly you can't go to someone's house for dinner and then sound them up and ask for the menu to include lots of Sirtfoods. Once again, neither of the books provides any suggestions for this scenario! I chose to go with approximately the same plan as the night before: small parts and my staying 2 glasses of red wine for the week! I just about managed to stick to my strategy, but it was really hard-- especially when the cheese course came out! And I was really sad not to be able to attempt either of the 2 whiskeys on offer at the end of the night

- DAY 14 SUNDAY

I had a bit more time on Sunday morning so decided to make the Sirtfood Pancakes, which need to have been Saturday's breakfast. These delicious pancakes were made with buckwheat flour, instead of wheat flour, and served with a delicious dark chocolate sauce, strawberries and walnuts. They were unbelievably great and rather the kids thought all their Christmases had come at when. My only grievance would be that the dish required 1 tablespoon of double cream and there were no other dishes that required double cream in the next few days, meaning the cream would have been lost ... if it hadn't been for the fact my kids and other half guaranteed to help me polish it off!

For Sunday lunch we all had the pittas once again, with more feta and this time lemon and coriander houmous-- likewise scrumptious and the kids delighted in selecting what to put in their pittas. For supper, we had the pizzas that we must have had on Saturday evening. Like with the pancakes, the pizzas were made using buckwheat flour. The tomato sauce has red onion in it too for added Sirtfood goodness. There are numerous concepts for toppings but I chose goats cheese, rocket, and chili... for me and me and my partner ... I let the kids pick what they wished to have and they plumped for cheddar cheese, mushrooms, peppers, and oregano. We all had enjoyable making and consuming the pizzas and it was a lovely thing to do as a family on a Sunday afternoon. And a beautiful end to week 2 of the Sirtfood Diet.

SIRTFOOD DIET WEEK 2: REFLECTIONS AND SUGGESTIONS

A DIET FOR FOODIES

Week 1 was quite nice, but in Week 2 the dishes got even much better: highlights have consisted of, that remarkable Sirtfood Chilli, the fantastic potato salad, those chocolate-covered pancakes, and the fantastic Sirtfood pizzas!-- and I've been looking ahead to what I prepare to cook next week, mostly from The Sirtfood Diet Recipe Book and the recipes are even better. With the possible exception of Week 1, this is absolutely a diet plan for foodies!

HEALTH BENEFITS

I haven't lost any weight this week. In truth I put a pound on, which is a bit unfortunate-- but hardly surprising given that today included a trip to dinner and a restaurant celebration! I have continued to experience all the other advantages of the Sirtfood Diet that I experienced in the very first week-- more so in truth now I am consuming effectively. I am feeling extremely perky, alert, and extremely favorable. I am likewise still sleeping like the proverbial baby. However, then I guess I should not be shocked given that I am feeding my body lots of very healthy foods, complete of minerals and vitamins, and not consuming any junk/processed food/ refined carbohydrates or sugar. I think possibly there is a lot to be said for the adage: you are what you eat!

PART SIZES

One of my gripes recently was the portion sizes appeared enormous. I haven't discovered that at all this week. I indicate they have been well huge, in a non-diety kind of way, but I've constantly been able to eat them and usually left the table sensation 'almost full' as you are expected to rather than starving or stuffed! Some of the meals have been so great I have wished I was allowed to have a more, mind! I have attempted very hard to stick to the recommended portion sizes and have primarily handled it!

VARIETY AND LEFTOVERS

The last week I got thoroughly fed up with kale, celery, and buckwheat in week 1. This week was so much better-- a lot more variety!

One grievance I would make this week is there was so much variety that things didn't get used up. I had leftover pittas that would have gone to waste if I had not rejigged things to ensure I utilized them up and remaining cream that thankfully my family ended up for me. It would also have been excellent if the meal plan had been written in a way that indicated you made extra of the suppers and used the leftovers up the next day for lunch, for that reason making my life simpler!

RESTAURANTS AND PARTIES

I truly tried to choose 3 weeks to do this diet where there were going to be relatively few social events, but my life is so hectic, there was never going to be a 3-week duration where absolutely nothing took place! One difficulty with this diet plan is it doesn't give you much aid with how to deal with restaurants and supper celebrations. It's a diet plan with a meal plan which says 'consume this on this day'.

LOOKING AHEAD TO WEEK 3 ...

Week 3 is more of the very same. In the very first book, 'The Sirtfood Diet' is precisely the same: the plan for weeks 2 and 3 are similar. Well, I figured that would make for a pretty dull article next week if I just did exactly the like today!

Instead I am going to use the next week to explore all the other options available in the second book: The Sirtfood Diet Recipe Book. I have read ahead and I am so delighted by some the recipes-- I'm anticipating attempting the Sirtfood Burger, Beef Bourguignon, Fajitas, Burritos, and Coq au Vin as well as a few family favorites like Chicken Korma and Spaghetti Bolognese-- all with a little Sirtfood twist! My only issue is, there may not be enough days in Week 3 to attempt them all out

➤

➢ SIRTFOOD DIET WEEK 3 SAMPLE

- DAY 15 MONDAY

Whilst I did wish to experiment with lots of brand-new recipes, I likewise desired to repeat some of my favorites too, so Monday I began out with among my absolute favorites from the week before the Sirt Muesli, with yogurt and mixed berries. Still absolutely delicious.

For lunch, I chose a brand-new dish from The Sirtfood Diet Recipe Book: The Tuna Nicoise Salad. This is a reasonably typical Nicoise salad, however, it does not include any potatoes and has been slight 'Sirtified' with the addition of celery, red onion, rocket, and parsley. I am not a big fan of hard-boiled eggs, so I had an avocado rather. This salad was so excellent. I was rather pleased I had half a tin of tuna leftover ... it meant I would just need to have it again the next day ... such a pity!

Well, I thought lunch was excellent, but dinner turned out to be even better. It was a Chicken Korma and I wasn't anticipating much, as I had been a bit disappointed by the previous week's curry. I was oh so wrong. It was so great. Even much better, I think, than my dish for chicken korma. And I like mine ... a lot! In reality, I would go as far as to state the Sirtfood Korma, or at least my variation of it, is probably the best korma I've ever eaten. It was truly basic to do too. I adapted the recipe a bit. (I simply can't assist myself! I have to streamline recipes!!) It's onions, garlic and ginger zoomed approximately make a paste. Diced chicken thighs are fried in the paste together with spices: turmeric, cumin, garam masala, cinnamon, and cardamoms. I then included coconut milk and simmered for 45 minutes. I included coriander leaves and served with it with buckwheat, although I'm sure this would go well with basmati rice too. This is set to end up being a Gargano family favorite for sure!

I was so complete of beans from my Chicken Korma that I decided it would be enjoyable to choose a run ... yes on one of the hottest nights of the year! Simply goes to show positive and energetic I've been feeling on this diet plan. Such behavior is not typical for me, I can ensure you!

And I have a sensation it won't stop now that I'm off the diet. A little benefit for consuming well all day and it stops me snacking on other, less healthy things !!

- DAY 16 TUESDAY

On Tuesday I went back to my other old favorite breakfast of yogurt with berries, cacao nibs, walnuts, and coconut flakes, which was as tasty as always. Another little practice I believe I'll be keeping up now my 3-week stint on the Sirtfood Diet is over

Sirtfood Breakfast of Yoghurt, Berries, Walnuts, Coconut Flakes and Cacao Nibs

It went so well with the salad-- specifically the tuna and the green beans. I do get the impression that apart from being full of Sirtfoods this diet plan is also fairly low carb.

Supper began out as a little bit of a disaster. I was planning to make the Kidney Bean Mole (a vegetarian variation of the Mexican classic-- for more about Mexican mole check out this post) Anyway, I discovered that I had failed to buy any kidneys beans ... surprisingly enough a key active ingredient in KIDNEY BEAN Mole, so I wound up having to use a tin of chickpeas which ended up being a fantastic idea (I do have them periodically) and the final dish tasted so incredible I had simply had to share it. You can discover the recipe for my Spicy Chickpea Stew here. (Well I had to relabel it for obvious factors!) This also went through several adjustments as quite apart from the kidney bean drama the component list was long and ... how shall I put this ... I couldn't be bothered! I did what I do best and streamlined it ... rather dramatically! The outcome was wonderful and rather a bit easier, so I actually would advise you to take a peek at the dish!

- DAY 17 WEDNESDAY

Well, I believed you may all be getting a little bored if I simply kept rotating in between the Sirtfood Muesli and the yogurt and fruit alternatives (I would not be at all bored as I like them both a lot!), so today I tried the fruit bowl-- another 'recipe' from the Sirtfood Diet Recipe Book. It was a fab mix of plums, apples, grapes, and my usual berries to have with walnuts and yogurt-- great enough but I believe I choose the 'just berries' option. I also missed my cacao nibs-- I simply enjoy those things!

Wednesday's lunch was a repeat of that fantastic potato salad with trout and watercress from recently. I slightly adjusted things this week by swapping among the trout fillets for avocado and utilizing a mix of rocket, spinach, and watercress rather than just plain watercress and it was so yummy. I can see this is going to be a routine lunch option for me. In truth, I likewise prepared it in for Thursday AND Sunday I like it so much! And it's so fast and simple to do.

Wednesday is my routine running night and constantly presents me with foodie difficulties. This week my husband and kids were consuming early and I would be consuming after my run. I desired something that would be extremely simple to reheat after my run (when I am in no mood for cooking!).

Like the Sirtfood Chilli Con carne last week, this is the best kind of food for this situation. The Sirtfood Bolognese recipe is a fairly common Bolognese recipe and features lots of Sirtfoods: celery, red wine, cocoa, olive oil and parsley (well really the dish calls for basil, but my basil had gone off and so I substituted with parsley). For the full Sirtfood result you can serve it with buckwheat pasta however I'm scared I went for basic white spaghetti-- well I had just been for a run so I figured I was permitted a few additional carbohydrates!

- DAY 18 THURSDAY.

My other fun activity for Wednesday was whipping up a batch of Sirtfood Granola for my breakfast on Thursday. The Sirtfood Granola is jam packed with yummy Sirtfoods: buckwheat flakes, cacao nibs, walnuts, as well as lots of other nuts and seeds and even turmeric which gives the granola a slightly yellow color and a tip of spice. Absolutely one I'll be having once again-- which is a great thing as it does make rather a large quantity-- and I only made half the recommended quantity!!

Thursday's lunch was the trout, watercress, and potato salad again once again then for dinner I made the Sirtfood Coq au Vin.

- DAY 19 FRIDAY.

Well Friday started with the lovely Sirtfood Granola again and then I decided to make the Sirtfood Super Salad again for lunch. This time I had it with some lovely soft goat's cheese that I had leftover from doing the pizzas last Sunday.

Friday supper required to be both versatile and fast. Quick since Friday is the kids' swimming lesson and we do not get home till nearly 6 and versatile because I was going for a run and so I wouldn't be consuming till later on. I chose to go with the Kidney Bean Burritos, however, adjust it slightly to make things quicker, turning it into more of a Kidney Bean Chilli and serving it with rice. It was pretty incredible, though, and not all that various from my Quick Beany Chilli, which is a company household favorite. And it went down very perfectly with a glass of red wine-- the very first of the 3 per week I am enabled on the Sirtfood Diet. After almost a week of abstinence, it decreased effectively undoubtedly!

Running at 7 pm always presents me with a bit of a challenge as to what to consume ahead of time. I obviously can't consume a full dinner at 6.30 with the kids, however, I truly need a little something to give me adequate energy for my run or I 'd slump. The response is a perfect little Sirtfood snack of 2 Medjool dates and a handful of walnuts. Much and completely tasty simpler to work up than a batch of Sirtfood Bites at brief notification!

- DAY 20 SATURDAY.

For breakfast on Saturday, I decided for granola and berries however this time decided have a pot of Coyo with it. Coyo is a vegan yogurt alternative made from coconut milk rather of dairy milk, resulting in an excellent tasting dairy and soy-free yogurt that is also gluten-free and included sugar-free too (though undoubtedly there is a bit of natural sugar from the coconut-- 1.9 g per 100g apparently), I truly liked the taste, but it was a bit of an odd texture: kind of the texture of goat's cheese, or as my other half less kindly put it-- Polyfilla!

Saturday lunch was those beautiful Sirtfood pittas again. The kids had great deals of enjoyable comprising their pittas from a variety of different ingredients. I do like lunches and dinners like that when the kids get to choose what to eat. They enjoy it and I do not get any 'I don't like that' arguments! I have a rule that they need to have 1 protein product (cheese or ham) and 2 salad products (from a choice of lettuce/cucumber/tomatoes/ avocado/rocket) and at least one pitta (or roll or piece of French bread, if I am not doing the Sirtfood diet) and the rest depends on them.

Dinner was one I 'd been looking forward to all week ... Beef Bourguignon-- a big favorite of mine. And in reality, the recipe is not very different from my own Beef Bourguignon recipe. The primary distinction being the addition of celery and carrots, and utilizing red onions rather of shallots. It was expected to be served with mashed potatoes and kale, however, I did it with new potatoes and green beans as I had actually some left over from the Coq au Vin and also it made the (admittedly rather wintery) stew seem a lot more summery. Needless to say, it was really tasty undoubtedly, and obviously, I had my 3rd and 2nd glasses of wine from my weekly quota with it!

I have been reflecting on different aspects of the Sirtfood Diet and one of the things I have noticed is there are absolutely no puddings on the diet plan. Certainly, you could have a couple of Sirtfood bites for a little pudding or the Lindt 85% Chocolate, but there are no actual pudding set up in.

- DAY 21 SUNDAY.

Well, it was Sirtfood Granola once again for breakfast today ... I desired to finish it up as it was my last day on the diet plan and the rest of my family didn't seem too keen on it! I believe probably because it is a lot less sweet than the other breakfast choices. I do tend to buy the healthier sounding cereals, but even a few of them have a horrible great deal of sugar in them! I have to state though, although the Sirtfood breakfasts have been beautiful, I have missed my usual breakfast of Shredded Wheat with milk and a little glass of orange juice! I will be having that tomorrow. Though I might simply be tempted to mix breakfast up a bit from now on and toss in the odd yogurt and berries or Sirtfood Muesli-- I might even attempt making my granola ... and I will certainly be making that chocolate porridge once again-- especially before another long Saturday run-- rocket fuel that stuff, I inform you!

Lunch was trout fillets once again with that beautiful potato salad, plus my favorite rocket/watercress/spinach mix and avocado too. I made this lunch again because I desired to share it with my family. I understood it would decrease well with them. Specifically, my other half, who loves this sort of food. My kids do too. Although I did provide them plain boiled potatoes as I understand they would not have been eager on all the 'amusing stuff' in the potato salad and, needless to state they did not have any avocado! They did hoover up good quantities of trout, potatoes and salad leaves.

Well that was what my family ate and what I was supposed to consume, however, I wound up opting for a run at lunch break, so had 2 banana muffins (approximately based upon my banana bread dish-- not extremely sirtfood, although they did include dark chocolate chips !!) to keep me going and when I got back I didn't feel hungry and after that, it was almost dinner time, so I wound up not having lunch at all.

And our last Sirtfood supper was Chicken Fajitas! A terrific way to end the diet. I always enjoy fajitas as it is enjoyable to put all the things in the middle and let everyone help themselves. I went for wholemeal tortillas, instead of white ones, given that this is what the recipe recommended and I was really happy with them. A nice little swap to make the supper a little more healthy and they tasted fantastic. May do that again in the future! The fajitas were served with guacamole, rocket, salsa, and cheddar cheese. I utilized my recipes for the guacamole and salsa as I didn't like the noise of the dishes in the book and reality the chicken fajita recipe wasn't that much different from mine, but I followed the recipe in the book and it turned out fantastic.

SIRTFOOD DIET WEEK 3: REFLECTIONS AND SUGGESTIONS

I have been musing on different aspects of the diet plan over the last couple of weeks. If you wish to look at my numerous thoughts on the Sirtfood diet plan do have a look at my reports on week 1 and week 2, but as I have now finished the diet I thought it would be helpful to give my general reflections on the diet as a whole and address 2 important concerns: did it work and would I suggest it?

DID THE SIRTFOOD DIET WORK?

By the end of the diet, I had lost a grand overall of 6lb. Not huge, but not insignificant for 3 weeks dieting either. The vast majority of that weight loss took place in the first week.

I do not think the second and third weeks are pointless by any methods. Firstly the meals are tasty and jam loaded with healthy ingredients: lots of fruit and veg, whole grains, nuts, seeds, pulses, healthy fats and lean protein, which can only have been a good idea for my body and far much better for me than some faddy diet plans that include a lot of processed foods and concealed sugars.

The diet plan is likewise low in sugar (apart from naturally happening fruit sugar) and I believe has served a fantastic purpose in re-educating my taste buds/ habits to a healthier method of consuming: no-calorie beverages (including lots of water and natural teas), essentially no snacking, no puddings (well apart from those two saucy squares of chocolate), less alcohol and smaller sized portions. All the things I know are healthy and good for me, however, I do not always do. However, 2 weeks of eating like that have encouraged me that I can do it and I believe I'm much more most likely to continue in that vein.

In this sirtfood diet book, the authors discuss how they observed that participants in their trials not only slimmed down in fat however likewise gained muscle (typically when dieting, individuals lose weight in muscle, which is not desirable as loss of muscle makes it even harder to burn calories and so move fat). Usually, participants on the Sirtfood diet plan seemed to lose only 5lb in weight, however, in fact, they got 2lb in muscle. Their total fat loss was 7lb.

My stomach is MUCH flatter than it was 3 weeks back and I certainly have less 'unsteady bits'. I want I 'd determined it at the start of the diet plan so I could provide you an actual concrete number, however, I reckon, going on belt notches, I've lost a couple of inches-- which I'm truly chuffed with.

The advantages of this diet go far beyond inches and pounds lost. Can't promise you it was down to the Sirtfood Diet but it at least points in the best direction!

I believe the most concrete and most remarkable thing of all for me in doing this diet has been the result of the quality of my sleep. It has changed quite considerably. Before doing the diet, I was the sort of person who usually tossed and turned A LOT throughout the night and semi awakened or perhaps correctly awakened a few times per night, often seeming like I 'd not slept at all. On the Sirtfood Diet, I have slept so well-- that type of sleep where you go to sleep and wake up which's it-- no tossing or turning or waking in between. I can't promise this will work for everybody, however, if you do battle with getting quality sleep, it may be worth trying!

I think this diet plan has taught me above all that what you put in your body truly does have a result on how you feel, how you sleep, and naturally your weight and body structure. If you put rubbish into your body, you can't be shocked when you feel rubbish. I have never felt so brilliant eyed and bushy-tailed as I have on this diet plan.

NOTE: YOU CAN FOLLOW MY PERSONAL EXPERIENCE, JUST SCROLL DOWN TO THE RECIPES SECTION AND CHOOSE THE RECIPES FOR EACH DAY.

GOOD LUCK

MEAL PLANNING

The charming feature of doing the Sirtfood Diet is that you get a few weeks off meal planning. This is something that often takes me half an hour or more on a Monday night. It is really lovely just to have a strategy and just two options to pick from each day.

SHOPPING

The majority of the active ingredients are truly simple to purchase in a regular supermarket: things like kale, celery, parsley, chilies, even buckwheat (groats) I discovered in my local Tesco. However, there are a couple of things which a bit difficult to get hold of. The things I discovered hard to get were:

Coconut Flakes-- I discovered these in my local health food shop, however, you could sub in desiccated coconut.

Buckwheat Pasta-- Again my regional health food store came up trumps, however, you could use brown rice pasta or simply wholemeal pasta if you didn't wish to make the trek.

Buckwheat Flakes/Puffs-- I discovered these on Amazon but they cost a fortune! I eventually found the flakes in Waitrose and chose just to get these and switch the puffs for flakes in the dish. If you can't get hold of them, porridge oats would most likely do as a substitute.

Matcha Green Tea-- This I could just discover on Amazon-- I bought this one. It cost £ 12 and the tub is tiny!! It's for the green juice and to be sincere, if I was doing the diet once again, I most likely wouldn't bother, but instead consume lots of Pukka Herbs Supreme Matcha Green tea, which I discovered in Tesco and has a percentage of matcha in it and tastes terrific. Quickly the best green tea I have attempted, without any bitter aftertaste.

Buckwheat Noodles-- I could not discover 100% buckwheat ones in Tesco but found them in Waitrose and the organic food store. If you don't fancy the trek, I 'd get the wheat and buckwheat ones or simply sub in typical noodles.

Lovage-- I drew an overall blank here. Goodness understands where you can get this from. I simply did without, or in some cases replaced with parsley.

MONEY

The problem with all these specialty items is that they are quite pricey (particularly the matcha tea-- ouch!), which makes this diet a bit difficult to do if you are on a tight spending plan. This diet plan was at first trialed in a unique London health club and expense was most likely not an issue there. Apart from a few specialty products, the bulk of the active ingredients are fairly typical and not too expensive. If you are on a tight budget it may be worth generally doing the veggie/vegan dishes which tend to concentrate on cheap veggies and staples such as beans, lentils, and buckwheat and miss out on out and/or replace a few of the more expensive ingredients, like buckwheat noodles and matcha tea.

JUICER

If you desire to make the juice, there is no way around this, except to get a juicer, which can be pretty expensive. The one I found and have been happily utilizing is the Philips HR1867/21 Viva Collection Juicer and, although the retail rate is £ 110, it is currently on the deal. You may just not desire to shell out on an expensive piece of kit just to decide the diet is not for you.

Sadly, you can't simply blitz the ingredients in a blender/food processor. Or at least I attempted when I was preparing for the diet and it was a disgusting green sludge! And my online research study suggests I am not the only one to discover this. You might attempt sieving the sludge or using a muslin/nut bag to squeeze the juice out, however, that does sound like rather a palaver or you might turn the green juice into a salad as I did on Wednesday (see below for the dish).

BEVERAGES

Essentially your options are water, green tea, black coffee, and black tea (and 2-3 little glasses of red wine in weeks 2 & 3). I constantly discover it amazing simply how numerous calories are hidden in drinks, which do not even fill you up!

I utilized to be awful with drinks-- juice, hot chocolate, and alcohol were my particular weak point. I've been working on this little vice for simply over a year and so I didn't discover it too awful. Plus, I am an overall coffee nut and I enjoy green tea (specifically the Pukka Herbs Supreme Matcha Green), but if you are utilized to drinking lots of calorie-filled drinks it might be worth lowering before starting this diet plan, so it's not excessive of a shock.

And though that was often coffee and green tea, it was more often water that I truly fancied. I also allowed myself camomile and peppermint tea when I got a bit bored of water and didn't want any more caffeine.

VEGAN OPTIONS

Every day has a meat/fish option and a veggie/vegan choice. I discovered this quite valuable when meal preparation. I selected the one I liked the sound of many. The veggie/vegan choices likewise do tend to be simpler-- excellent for hectic days! And they are also more affordable-- my mix and match approach certainly lowered the cost of my shopping significantly.

KIDS (AND HUSBAND!).

I offered them a regular breakfast while I had a green juice. They were at school (work) on the days when I had green juice for lunch and for the lunches and suppers they were around for, they just had the same as me. Mostly they were happy, and I did choose carefully, however, they did get a bit fed up of buckwheat and kale, but then so did I!

The book states specifically that it is OK to give the kids the meals, but not the juice-- to be truthful I 'd be rather surprised if you could find a kid who would drink the juice !! But I believe a lot of kids would not be as accommodating as mine. , if your kids (or other half!) are a bit fussier than my own you may discover you need to prepare separate meals and/or make some adjustments, such as alternative carbs (if they are not fans of buckwheat) or alternative veggies (if they are not fans of celery and kale).

Are you enjoying this book? I'd be glad to know what you think. Leave a short review on Amazon. Thank you

THE SIRTFOOD DIET RECIPES

TURMERIC CHICKEN & KALE SALAD WITH HONEY LIME DRESSING

Prep time

20 mins

Cook time

10 mins

Total time

30 mins

Notes: If preparing ahead of time, dress the salad 10 minutes before serving. Chicken can be replaced with beef mince, chopped prawns or fish. Vegetarians could use chopped mushrooms or cooked quinoa.

Dish out s: 2

Things needed

For the chicken

* 1 teaspoon ghee or 1 table spoon coconut oil

* ½ medium brown onion, diced

* 250-300 g / 9 oz. chicken mince or diced up chicken thighs

* 1 large garlic clove, finely diced

* 1 teaspoon turmeric powder

* 1teaspoon lime zest

* juice of ½ lime

* ½ teaspoon salt + pepper

For the salad

* 6 broccolini stalks or 2 cups of broccoli florets

* 2 tablespoons pumpkin seeds (pepitas)

* 3 large kale leaves, stems removed and chopped

* ½ avocado, sliced

* handful of fresh coriander leaves, chopped

* handful of fresh parsley leaves, chopped

For the dressing

* 3 tablespoons lime juice

* 1 small garlic clove, finely diced or grated

* 3 tablespoons extra-virgin olive oil (I used 1 tablespoons avocado oil and * 2 tablespoons EVO)

*1 teaspoon raw honey

* ½ teaspoon wholegrain or Dijon mustard

* ½ teaspoon sea salt and pepper

Steps

1. First heat the ghee or coconut oil in a small frying pan over medium-high first heat. Include the onion and sauté on medium first heat for 4-5 minutes, until golden. Include the chicken mince and garlic and stir for 2-3 minutes over medium-high first heat, breaking it apart.

2. Include the turmeric, lime zest, lime juice, salt and pepper and cook, stirring frequently, for a further 3-4 minutes. Set the cooked mince aside.

3. While the chicken is cooking, bring a small saucepan of water to boil. Include the broccolini and cook for 2 minutes. Rinse under cold water and cut into 3-4 pieces each.

4. Include the pumpkin seeds to the frying pan from the chicken and toast over medium first heat

for 2 minutes, stirring frequently to prevent burning. Season with a little salt. Set aside. Raw pumpkin seeds are also fine to use.

5. Place chopped kale in a salad bowl and pour over the dressing. Using your hands, toss and massage the kale with the dressing. This will soften the kale, kind of like what citrus juice does to fish or beef carpaccio – it 'cooks' it slightly.

6. Finally toss through the cooked chicken, broccolini, fresh herbs, pumpkin seeds and avocado slices.

BUCKWHEAT NOODLES WITH CHICKEN KALE & MISO DRESSING

Dish out s: 2

Things needed

For the noodles

* 2-3 handfuls of kale leaves (removed from the stem and roughly cut)

* 150 g / 5 oz buckwheat noodles (100% buckwheat, no wfirst heat)

* 3-4 shiitake mushrooms, sliced

* 1 teaspoon coconut oil or ghee

* 1 brown onion, finely diced

* 1 medium free-range chicken breast, sliced or diced

* 1 long red chilli, thinly sliced (seeds in or out depending on how hot you like it)

* 2 large garlic cloves, finely diced

* 2-3 tablespoons Tamari sauce (gluten-free soy sauce)

For the miso dressing

* 1½ tablespoon fresh organic miso

* 1 tablespoon Tamari sauce

* 1 tablespoon extra-virgin olive oil

* 1 tablespoon lemon or lime juice

* 1 teaspoon sesame oil (optional)

Steps

1. Bring a medium saucepan of water to boil. Include the kale and cook for 1 minute, until

slightly wilted. Remove and set aside but reserve the water and bring it back to the boil. Include the soba noodles and cook according to the package steps (usually about 5 minutes). Rinse under cold water and set aside.

2. In the meantime, pan fry the shiitake mushrooms in a little ghee or coconut oil (about a teaspoon) for 2-3 minutes, until lightly browned on each side. Sprinkle with sea salt and set aside.

3. In the same frying pan, first heat more coconut oil or ghee over medium-high first heat. Sauté onion and chilli for 2-3 minutes and then include the chicken pieces. Cook 5 minutes over medium first heat, stirring a couple of times, then include the garlic, tamari sauce and a little splash of water. Cook for a further 2-3 minutes, stirring frequently until chicken is cooked through.

4. Finally, include the kale and soba noodles and toss through the chicken to warm up.

5.Mix the miso dressing and drizzle over the noodles right at the end of cooking, this way you will keep all those beneficial probiotics in the miso alive and active.

ASIAN KING PRAWN STIR-FRY WITH BUCKWHEAT NOODLES

Dish out 1

Things needed:

150g shelled raw king prawns, deveined

2 tea spoon tamari (you can use soy sauce if you are not avoiding gluten)

2 tea spoon extra virgin olive oil

75g soba (buckwheat noodles)

1 garlic clove, finely chopped

1 bird's eye chilli, finely chopped

1 tea spoon finely chopped fresh ginger

20g red onions, sliced

40g celery, trimmed and sliced

75g green beans, chopped

50g kale, roughly chopped

100ml chicken stock

5g lovage or celery leaves

Steps:

First heat a frying pan over a high first heat, then cook the prawns in 1 teaspoon of the tamari and 1 teaspoon of the oil for 2–3 minutes. Transfer the prawns to a plate. Wipe the pan out with kitchen paper, as you're going to use it again.

Cook the noodles in boiling water for 5–8 minutes or as directed on the packet. Drain and set aside.

Meanwhile, fry the garlic, chilli and ginger, red onion, celery, beans and kale in the remaining oil over a medium–high first heat for 2–3 minutes. Include the stock and bring to the boil, then simmer for a minute or two, until the vegetables are cooked but still crunchy.

Include the prawns, noodles and lovage/celery leaves to the pan, bring back to the boil then remove from the first heat and dish out .

BAKED SALMON SALAD WITH CREAMY MINT DRESSING-SIRTFOOD

340 calories - 3 of your SIRT 5 a day

Baking the salmon in the microwave makes this salad so simple.

Dispense s 1 - Ready in 20 minutes

Things required

1 salmon fillet (130g).

40g combined salad leaves.

40g young spinach leaves.

2 radishes, trimmed and thinly sliced.

5cm piece (50g) cucumber, cut into chunks.

2 spring onions, sliced and trimmed.

1 little handful (10g) parsley, roughly sliced.

For the dressing:

1 tea spoon low-fat mayo.

1 table spoon natural yogurt.

1 table spoon rice vinegar.

2 leaves mint, carefully sliced.

Salt and newly ground black pepper.

step.

1 Prefirst heat the microwave oven to 200 ° C (180 ° C fan/Gas

6). 2 Place the salmon fillet on a baking tray and bake for 16-- 18 minutes till simply cooked through. Eliminate from the microwave and reserved. The salmon is equally good hot or cold in the salad. Simply prepare skin side down and get rid of the salmon from the skin utilizing a fish slice after cooking if your salmon has skin. When prepared, it ought to slide off quickly.

3 In a little bowl, mix together the mayo, yogurt, rice wine vinegar, mint leaves and salt and pepper together and delegate represent at least 5 minutes to permit the.

tastes to establish.

4 Arrange the salad leaves and spinach on a serving plate and top with the radishes, cucumber, spring onions and parsley. Flake the prepared salmon onto the salad and drizzle the dressing over.

CHOC CHIP GRANOLA.

244 calories.

1/2 of your SIRT 5 a day.

Chocolate at breakfast! Make certain to dish out with a cup of green tea to give you a lot of SIRTs. If you choose, the rice malt syrup can be replaced with maple syrup.

Dispense s 8 - Ready in 30 minutes.

Things required.

200g jumbo oats.

50g pecans, approximately.

sliced.

3 table spoon light olive oil.

20g butter.

1 table spoon dark brown sugar.

2 table spoon rice malt syrup.

60g good-quality (70%).

dark chocolate chips.

step.

Pre first heat the microwave to 160 ° C (140 ° C fan/Gas 3). Line a large baking tray with a silicone sheet or baking parchment.

In a little non-stick pan, carefully first heat the olive oil, butter, brown sugar and rice malt syrup till the butter has actually melted and the sugar and syrup have actually dissolved. Pour the syrup over the oats and stir completely till the oats are totally covered.

Distribute the granola over the baking tray, spreading right into the corners. Leave clumps of mixture with spacing rather than an even spread. Bake in the microwave for 20 minutes till just tinged golden brown at the edges. Get rid of from the microwave oven and leave to cool on the tray entirely.

When cool, break up any bigger swellings on the tray with your fingers and after that blend in the chocolate chips. Scoop or put the granola into an airtight tub or jar. The granola will keep for a minimum of 2 weeks.

FRAGRANT ASIAN HOTPOT.

185 calories.

1 1/2 of you SIRT 5 a day.

Dish out s 2 - Ready in 15 minutes.

Things needed.

1 tea spoon tomato purée.

1 star anise, crushed (or 1/4 tea spoon ground anise).

Small handful (10g) parsley, stalks carefully chopped.

Little handful (10g) coriander, stalks finely sliced.

Juice of 1/2 lime.

500ml chicken stock, fresh or made with 1 cube.

1/2 carrot, peeled and cut into matchsticks.

50g broccoli, cut into little florets.

50g beansprouts.

100g raw tiger prawns.

100g company tofu, sliced.

50g rice noodles, prepared according to packet actions.

50g prepared water chestnuts, drained pipes.

20g sushi ginger, chopped.

1 table spoon good-quality miso paste.

Actions.

Location the tomato purée, star anise, parsley stalks, coriander stalks, lime juice and chicken stock in a big pan and bring to a simmer for 10 minutes.

Consist of the carrot, broccoli, prawns, tofu, noodles and water chestnuts and simmer gently up until the prawns are cooked through. Get rid of from the first heat and stir in the sushi ginger and miso paste.

Dispense sprinkled with the parsley and coriander leaves.

LAMB, BUTTERNUT SQUASH AND DATE TAGINE- SIRTFOOD RECIPES.

Preparation time 15 minutes.

Cook time 1 hour 15 minutes.

Total time 1 hour 30 mins.

Unbelievable warming Moroccan spices make this healthy tagine ideal for chilly autumn and winter nights. Dish out with buckwheat for an additional health kick!

Dispense: 4.

Things required.

2 tablespoons olive oil.

1 red onion, sliced.

2cm ginger, grated.

3 garlic cloves, grated or crushed.

1 teaspoon chilli flakes (or to taste).

2 teaspoons cumin seeds.

1 cinnamon stick.

2 teaspoons ground turmeric.

800g lamb neck fillet, cut into 2cm chunks.

1/2 teaspoon salt.

100g medjool dates, pitted and sliced.

400g tin sliced tomatoes, plus half a can of water.

500g butternut squash, sliced into 1cm cubes.

400g tin chickpeas, drained pipes.

2 tablespoons fresh coriander (plus additional for garnish).

Buckwheat, couscous, flatbreads or rice to dish out.

Method.

1. Pre first heat your microwave to 140C.

2. Drizzle about 2 tablespoons of olive oil into a large microwave ovenproof saucepan or cast iron casserole meal. Include the chopped onion and cook on a mild very first heat, with the cover on, for about 5 minutes, until the onions are softened but not brown.

Stir well and prepare for 1 more minute with the cover off. Include a splash of water if it gets too dry.

4. Next include in the lamb pieces. Stir well to coat the meat in the spices and onions and then consist of the salt, sliced dates, and tomatoes, plus about half a can of water (100-200ml).

5. Bring the tagine to the boil and then place the cover on and location in your prefirst heated microwave for 1 hour and 15 minutes.

6. Half an hour prior to the end of the cooking time, consist of in the chopped butternut squash and drained chickpeas. Stir everything together, put the lid back on and go back to the microwave

for the final 30 minutes of cooking.

7. When the tagine is ready, eliminate from the microwave and stir through the sliced coriander. Dispense with buckwheat, couscous, basmati or flatbreads rice.

Notes.

If you do not own an microwave ovenproof pan or cast iron casserole meal, simply prepare the tagine in a regular pan up till it has to go in the microwave and then transfer the tagine into a regular lidded casserole meal prior to putting in the microwave oven. Include on an extra 5 minutes cooking time to enable for the fact that the casserole meal will need extra time to first heat up.

PRAWN ARRABBIATA.

Dispense s 1.

Preparation time:

35-- 40 minutes.

Cooking time:

20-- 30 minutes.

Things required.

125-150 g Raw or cooked prawns (Ideally king prawns).

65 g Buckwheat pasta.

1 table spoon Extra virgin olive oil.

For arrabbiata sauce.

40 g Red onion, carefully chopped.

1 Garlic clove, finely chopped.

30 g Celery, finely sliced.

1 Bird's eye chilli, carefully sliced.

1 teaspoon Dried combined herbs.

1 tea spoon Extra virgin olive oil.

2 table spoon White white wine (optional).

400 g Tinned chopped tomatoes.

1 table spoon Chopped parsley.

Approach.

Fry the onion, garlic, celery and chilli and dried herbs in the oil over a medium-- low first heat for

1-- 2 minutes. Turn the very first heat up to medium, consist of the red wine and cook for 1 minute.

2. While the sauce is cooking bring a pan of water to the boil and cook the pasta according to the package actions. When cooked to your taste, drain, toss with the olive oil and keep in the pan up until needed.

3. If you are utilizing raw prawns include them to the sauce and cook for an additional 3-- 4 minutes, until they have turned opaque and pink, consist of the parsley and dispense. If you are using cooked prawns include them with the parsley, bring the sauce to the boil and dish out.

4. Include the prepared pasta to the sauce, mix thoroughly however gently and dispense.

TURMERIC BAKED SALMON

Dispense: 1

Preparation time:

10-- 15 minutes

Cooking time:

10 minutes

Things needed

125-150 g Skinned Salmon

1 tea spoon Extra virgin olive oil

1 tea spoon Ground turmeric

1/4 Juice of a lemon

For the spicy celery

1 tea spoon Extra virgin olive oil

40 g Red onion, finely chopped

60 g Tinned green lentils

1 Garlic clove, carefully sliced

1 cm Fresh ginger, carefully chopped

1 Bire's eye chilli, carefully chopped

150 g Celery, cut into 2cm lengths

1 tea spoon Mild curry powder

130 g Tomato, cut into 8 wedges

100 ml Chicken or vegetable stock

1 table spoon Chopped parsley

Approach

Heat the microwave oven to 200C/ gas mark 6.

Start with the spicy celery. Heat a frying pan over a
medium-- low first heat, include the olive oil, then
the onion, garlic, celery, ginger and chilli. Fry gently
for 2-- 3 minutes or until softened but not
coloured, then include the curry powder and cook
for an additional minute.

Include the tomatoes then the stock and lentils and
simmer carefully for 10 minutes. You might want to
increase or reduce the cooking time depending
upon how crispy you like your celery.

Mix the turmeric, oil and lemon juice and rub over
the salmon. # Place on a baking tray and cook for 8-
- 10 minutes.

To end up, stir the parsley through the celery and
dish outwith the salmon.

CORONATION CHICKEN SALAD-SIRTFOOD RECIPES

Dish out s 1

Preparation time: 5 minutes

Things required

75 g Natural yoghurt

Juice of 1/4 of a lemon

1 tea spoon Coriander, sliced

1 tea spoon Ground turmeric

1/2 tea spoon Mild curry powder

100 g Cooked chicken breast, cut into bite-sized pieces

6 Walnut halves, finely chopped

1 Medjool date, carefully sliced

20 g Red onion, diced

1 Bird's eye chilli

40 g Rocket, to dish out

Approach

Mix the yoghurt, lemon juice, coriander and spices together in a bowl. Include all the staying things required and meal outon a bed of the rocket.

BAKED POTATOES WITH SPICY CHICKPEA STEW

Prep time

10 minutes

Prepare time

1 hour

Dispense s 4-6

Type Of Mexican Mole satisfies North African Tagine, this Spicy Chickpea Stew is unbelievably tasty and makes a fantastic topping for baked potatoes, plus it just occurs to be vegetarian, vegan, gluten complimentary and dairy complimentary. And it includes chocolate.

Things needed

4-6 baking potatoes, punctured all over

2 tablespoons olive oil

2 red onions, finely sliced

4 cloves garlic, grated or crushed

2cm ginger, grated

1/2 -2 teaspoons chilli flakes (depending on how hot you like things).

2 tablespoons cumin seeds.

2 tablespoons turmeric.

Splash of water.

2 x 400g tins sliced tomatoes.

2 tablespoons unsweetened cocoa powder (or cacao).

If you prefer) consisting of the chickpea water DON'T DRAIN!!

2 yellow peppers (or whatever colour you prefer!), 2 x 400g tins chickpeas (or kidney beans, sliced into bitesize pieces.

2 tablespoons parsley plus additional for garnish.

Salt and pepper to taste (optional).

Side salad (optional).

Method.

Prefirst heat the microwave to 200C, meanwhile you can prepare all your things required.

When the microwave is hot sufficient location your baking potatoes in the microwave and cook for 1 hour or until they are done how you like them.

When the potatoes are in the microwave, position the olive oil and chopped red onion in a big broad pan and cook carefully, with the lid on for 5 minutes, till the onions are not brown however soft.

Remove the cover and include the garlic, chilli, ginger and cumin. Cook for a more minute on a low first heat, then consist of the turmeric and a really small splash of water and cook for another minute, taking care not to let the pan get too dry.

Next, include in the tomatoes, cocoa powder (or cacao), chickpeas (consisting of the chickpea water) and yellow pepper. Bring to the boil, then simmer on a low very first heat for 45 minutes till the sauce is thick and unctuous (but do not let it burn!). The stew must be done at roughly the same time as the potatoes.

Stir in the 2 tablespoons of parsley, and some salt and pepper if you wish, and meal out the stew on top of the baked potatoes, maybe with a basic side salad.

GRAPE AND MELON JUICE-SIRTFOOD RECIPES.

125 calories.

2 of your SIRT 5 a day.

Dish out s 1 - Ready in 2 minutes.

Components.

1/2 cucumber, peeled if preferred, halved, seeds got rid of and roughly chopped.

30g young spinach leaves, stalks got rid of.

100g red seedless grapes.

100g cantaloupe melon, peeled, deseeded and cut into pieces.

1 Blend together in a juicer or blender up until smooth.

KALE AND RED ONION DHAL WITH BUCKWHEAT-SIRTFOOD.

Prep time 5 minutes.

Cook time 25 mins.

Overall time 30 minutes.

Dish out:4.

Delicious and extremely healthy this Kale and Red Onion Dhal with Buckwheat is fast and simple to make and naturally gluten totally free, dairy totally free, vegetarian and vegan.

 THINGS NEEDED.

1 tablespoon olive oil.

1 little red onion, sliced.

3 garlic cloves, grated or squashed.

2 cm ginger, grated.

1 birds eye chilli, deseeded and carefully chopped (more if you like things hot!).

2 teaspoons turmeric.

2 teaspoons garam masala.

160g red lentils.

400ml coconut milk.

200ml water.

100g kale (or spinach would be a fantastic option).

160g buckwheat (or brown rice).

STEPS.

1. Location the olive oil in a large, deep saucepan and consist of the sliced onion. Cook on a low very first heat, with the lid on for 5 minutes up until softened.

2. Consist of the garlic, chilli and ginger and cook for 1 more minute.

3. Include the turmeric, garam masala and a splash of water and cook for 1 more minute.

4. Consist of the red lentils, coconut milk, and 200ml water (do this simply by half filling the coconut milk can with water and tipping it into the pan).

5. Mix everything together thoroughly and prepare for 20 minutes over a carefully first heat with the lid on. If the dhal starts to stick, stir periodically and

consist of a bit more water.

6. After 20 minutes include the kale, stir completely and change the cover, cook for a further 5 minutes (1-2 minutes if you utilize spinach instead!).

About 15 minutes prior to the curry is all set, place the buckwheat in a medium saucepan and consist of plenty of boiling water. Bring the water back to the boil and cook for 10 minutes (or a bit longer if you prefer your buckwheat softer.

CHARGRILLED BEEF WITH A RED WINE JUS, ONION RINGS, GARLIC KALE AND HERB ROASTED POTATOES-SIRTFOOD RECIPES.

THINGS NEEDED:

100g potatoes, peeled and cut into 2cm dice.

1 table spoon extra virgin olive oil.

5g parsley, carefully sliced.

50g red onion, sliced into rings.

50g kale, sliced.

1 garlic clove, carefully chopped.

120-- 150g x 3.5cm-thick beef fillet steak or 2cm-thick sirloin steak.

40ml red white wine.

150ml beef stock.

1 tea spoon tomato purée.

1 tea spoon cornflour, liquified in 1 table spoon water.

ACTIONS:

First heat the microwave to 220ºC/ gas 7.

Location the potatoes in a saucepan of boiling water, bring back to the boil and cook for 4-- 5 minutes, then drain. Location in a roasting tin with 1 teaspoon of the oil and roast in the hot microwave oven for 35-- 45 minutes.

Fry the onion in 1 teaspoon of the oil over a medium first heat for 5-- 7 minutes, until soft and well caramelised. Fry the garlic gently in 1/2 teaspoon of oil for 1 minute, up until soft but not coloured. Include the kale and fry for a further 1-- 2 minutes, till tender.

First heat an microwave ovenproof fry pan over a high first heat up until smoking cigarettes. Cover the meat in 1/2 a teaspoon of the oil and fry in the hot pan over a medium-- high first heat according to how you like your meat done.If you like your meat medium it would be better to sear the meat and then move the pan to a microwave set at 220ºC/ gas 7 and finish the cooking that method for the prescribed times.

Eliminate the meat from the pan and set aside to rest. Consist of the red wine to the hot pan to bring up any meat residue. Bubble to decrease the red wine by half, until syrupy and with a concentrated taste.

Consist of the stock and tomato purée to the steak pan and give the boil, then include the cornflour paste to thicken your sauce, including it a little at a time until you have your desired consistency. Stir in any of the juices from the rested steak and dispense with the roasted potatoes, kale, onion rings and red wine sauce.

KALE AND BLACKCURRANT SMOOTHIE.

86 calories.

1-- 1/2 of your SIRT 5 a day.

Dispense s 2 - Ready in 3 minutes.

Things needed.

2 tea spoon honey.

1 cup newly made green tea.

10 infant kale leaves, stalks eliminated.

1 ripe banana.

40 g blackcurrants, washed and stalks eliminated.

6 ice cubes.

Step.

Stir the honey into the warm green tea until dissolved. Whiz all the things needed together in a mixer until smooth. Dispense instantly.

BUCKWHEAT PASTA SALAD-SIRTFOOD RECIPES.

Dish out s 1.

Things required.

50g buckwheat pasta(cooked according to the packet steps).

large handful of rocket.

little handful of basil leaves.

8 cherry tomatoes, halved.

1/2 avocado, diced.

10 olives.

1 table spoon additional virgin olive oil.

20g pine nuts.

Carefully combine all the important things needed except the pine nuts and set up on a plate or in a bowl, then spread the pine nuts over the top.

GREEK SALAD SKEWERS-SIRTFOOD.

306 calories - 3.5 of your SIRT 5 a day.

Dish out s 2 - Ready in 10 minutes.

Things required.

2 wood skewers, soaked in water for 30 minutes prior to use.

8 large black olives.

8 cherry tomatoes.

1 yellow pepper, cut into 8 squares.

1/2 red onion, cut in half and separated into 8 pieces.

100g (about 10cm) cucumber, cut into 4 slices and halved.

100g feta, cut into 8 cubes.

For the dressing:

1 table spoon extra virgin olive oil.

Juice of 1/2 lemon.

1 tea spoon balsamic vinegar.

1/2 clove garlic, peeled and squashed.

Few leaves basil, carefully chopped (or 1/2 tea spoon dried blended herbs to change basil and oregano).

Few leaves oregano, carefully sliced.

Generous flavoring of salt and freshly ground black pepper.

Step.

Thread each skewer with the salad things needed in the order: olive, tomato, yellow pepper, red onion, cucumber, feta, tomato, olive, yellow pepper, red onion, cucumber, feta.

Location all the dressing things needed in a little bowl and blend together thoroughly. Put over the skewers.

KALE, EDAMAME, AND TOFU CURRY.

342 calories.

2 1/2 of your SIRT 5 a day.

A warming and wintry curry. Easy to keep either cooled or frozen for another day.

Dish out s 4 - Ready in 45 minutes.

Things needed.

1 table spoon rapeseed oil.

1 big onion, chopped.

4 cloves garlic, peeled and grated.

1 large thumb (7cm) fresh ginger, peeled and grated.

1 red chilli, deseeded and thinly sliced.

1/2 tea spoon ground turmeric.

1/4 tea spoon cayenne pepper.

1 tea spoon paprika.

1/2 tea spoon ground cumin.

1 tea spoon salt.

250g dried red lentils.

1 litre boiling water.

50g frozen soya edamame beans.

200g company tofu, chopped into cubes.

2 tomatoes, approximately sliced.

Juice of 1 lime.

200g kale leaves, stalks eliminated and torn.

Action.

Include the onion and cook for 5 minutes prior to including the garlic, chilli and ginger and cooking for a further 2 minutes. Stir through before including the red lentils and stirring once again.

Put in the boiling water and bring to a hearty simmer for 10 minutes, then minimize the very first heat and cook for a further 20-30 minutes till the curry has a thick '- porridge' consistency.

Consist of the soya beans, tofu and tomatoes and cook for a further 5 minutes. Consist of the lime juice and kale leaves and cook until the kale is simply tender.

CHOCOLATE CUPCAKES WITH MATCHA ICING.

234 calories - 1 of your SIRT 5 a day.

Simply awesome!

MAKES 12 - READY IN 35 MINUTES.

Things required.

150g self-raising flour.

200g caster sugar.

60g cocoa.

1/2 tea spoon salt.

1/2 tea spoon great espresso coffee, decaf if chosen.

120ml milk.

1/2 tea spoon vanilla extract.

50ml grease.

1 egg.

120ml boiling water.

For the icing:

50g butter, at space temperature.

50g icing sugar.

1 table spoon matcha green tea powder.

1/2 tea spoon vanilla bean paste.

50g soft cream cheese.

Actions.

- Prefirst heat the microwave oven to 180C/160C fan. Line a cupcake tin with paper or silicone cake cases.

- Place the flour, sugar, espresso, cocoa and salt powder in a large bowl and mix thoroughly.

- Include the milk, vanilla extract, veggie oil and egg to the dry things required and utilize an electric mixer to beat till well combined. Utilize a high speed to beat for a more minute to include air to the batter.

- Spoon the batter evenly in between the cake cases. Bake in the microwave oven for 15-18 minutes, up until the mix bounces back when tapped.

Include the matcha powder and vanilla and stir once again. Include the cream cheese and beat till smooth.

SESAME CHICKEN SALAD.

304 cals - 3.5 of your SIRT 5 a day.

A uncommon and tasty salad.

Dispense s 2 - Ready in 12 minutes.

Things required.

1 table spoon sesame seeds.

1 cucumber, peeled, cut in half lengthways, deseeded with a teaspoon and sliced.

100g child kale, roughly chopped.

60g pak choi, extremely carefully shredded.

1/2 red onion, really finely sliced.

Large handful (20g) parsley, chopped.

150g prepared chicken, shredded.

For the dressing:

1 table spoon additional virgin olive oil.

1 tea spoon sesame oil.

Juice of 1 lime.

1 tea spoon clear honey.

2 tea spoon soy sauce.

1 Toast the sesame seeds in a dry frying pan for 2 minutes up until lightly browned and aromatic. Transfer to a plate to cool.

2 In a little bowl, mix together the olive oil, sesame oil, lime honey, soy and juice sauce to make the dressing.

3 Place the cucumber, kale, pak choi, red onion and parsley in a big bowl and gently mix together. Put over the dressing and blend again.

4 Distribute the salad in between two plates and

top with the shredded chicken. Sprinkle over the sesame seeds simply before serving.

SIRTFOOD MUSHROOM SCRAMBLE EGGS.

Things needed.

2 eggs.

1 tea spoon ground turmeric.

1 teaspoon mild curry powder.

20g kale, roughly sliced.

1 tea spoon additional virgin olive oil.

1/2 bird's eye chilli, very finely sliced.

handful of button mushrooms, very finely sliced.

5g parsley, carefully chopped.

optional Include a seed mixture as a topper and some Rooster Sauce for taste.

Actions.

Mix the turmeric and curry powder and consist of a little water until you have achieved a light paste.

Steam the kale for 2-- 3 minutes.

Heat the oil in a frying pan over a medium very first heat and fry the chilli and mushrooms for 2-- 3 minutes up until they have actually begun to brown and soften.

FRAGRANT CHICKEN BREAST WITH KALE, RED ONION, AND SALSA-SIRTFOOD RECIPES SIRTFOOD RECIPES.

Things needed:

120g skinless, boneless chicken breast.

2 tea spoon ground turmeric.

juice of 1/4 lemon.

1 table spoon additional virgin olive oil.

50g kale, chopped.

20g red onion, sliced.

1 tea spoon chopped fresh ginger.

50g buckwheat.

Steps:

To make the salsa, remove the eye from the tomato and slice it really finely, taking care to keep as much of the liquid as possible. Blend with the chilli, capers, parsley and lemon juice. You might put everything in the end however a blender outcome is a bit different.

First heat the microwave oven to 220ºC/ gas 7. Marinate the chicken breast in 1 teaspoon of the turmeric, a little oil and the lemon juice. Leave for 5-- 10 minutes.

Very first heat an microwave ovenproof frying pan until hot, then include the marinated chicken and cook for a minute approximately on each side, up until pale golden, then transfer to the microwave (put on a baking tray if your pan isn't microwave ovenproof) for 8-- 10 minutes or till prepared through. Eliminate from the microwave, cover with foil and leave to rest for 5 minutes before serving.

Prepare the kale in a steamer for 5 minutes. Fry the red onions and the ginger in a little oil, up until soft however not coloured, then consist of the prepared kale and fry for another minute.

Cook the buckwheat according to the packet actions with the staying teaspoon of turmeric. Dish outalongside the chicken, vegetables and salsa.

SMOKED SALMON OMELETTE-.

Try this simple and quick Sirtfood dish packed with flavour and goodness.

Dispense s:1.

Preparation time:5-- 10 minutes.

Things needed.

2 Medium eggs.

100 g Smoked salmon, sliced.

1/2 tea spoon Capers.

10 g Rocket, chopped.

1 teaspoon Parsley, sliced.

1 tea spoon Extra virgin olive oil.

Method.

Split the eggs into a bowl and blend well. Include the salmon, capers, rocket and parsley.

Very first heat the olive oil in a non-stick fry pan up until hot however not cigarette smoking. Consist of the egg mix and, using a spatula or fish piece, move the mix around the pan until it is even. Reduce the first heat and let the omelette cook through. Slide the spatula around the edges and roll up or fold the omelette in half to dispense.

GREEN TEA SMOOTHIE.

183 calories.

1 of your SIRT 5 a day.

This super-healthy smoothie utilizes matcha powder, which is an extremely concentrated Japanese green tea. It can be discovered in specialist Asian or tea shops.

Dispense s 2 - Ready in 3 minutes.

Things required.

2 ripe bananas.

250 ml milk.

2 tea spoon matcha green tea powder.

1/2 tea spoon vanilla bean paste (not extract) or a little scrape of the seeds from a vanilla pod.

6 ice cubes.

2 tea spoon honey.

Just mix all the important things required together in a blender and dish outin 2 glasses.

SIRT FOOD MISO MARINATED COD WITH STIR-FRIED GREENS & SESAME-SIRTFOOD RECIPES.

DISH OUT.

THINGS NEEDED.

20g miso.

1 table spoon mirin.

1 tablespoon extra virgin olive oil.

200g skinless cod fillet.

20g red onion, sliced.

40g celery, sliced.

1 garlic clove, finely sliced.

1 bird's eye chilli, finely sliced.

1 tea spoon finely chopped fresh ginger.

60g green beans.

50g kale, approximately sliced.

1 tea spoon sesame seeds.

5g parsley, roughly chopped.

1 table spoon tamari.

30g buckwheat.

1 tea spoon ground turmeric.

STEPS.

Mix the miso, mirin and 1 teaspoon of the oil. Rub all over the cod and delegate marinate for 30 minutes. Heat the microwave oven to 220ºC/ gas 7.

Bake the cod for 10 minutes.

Include the onion and stir-fry for a few minutes, then consist of the celery, garlic, chilli, ginger, green beans and kale. You might require to consist of a little water to the pan to help the cooking process.

Prepare the buckwheat according to the packet steps with the turmeric for 3 minutes.

Consist of the sesame seeds, parsley and tamari to the stir-fry and meal outwith the greens and fish.

RASPBERRY AND BLACKCURRANT JELLY.

76 calories.

2 of your SIRT 5 a day.

Making a jelly beforehand is an excellent way to prepare the fruit so that it is all set to consume first thing in the early morning.

Dish out s 2 - Ready in 15 minutes + setting time.

Things needed.

100g raspberries, cleaned.

2 leaves gelatin.

100g blackcurrants, cleaned and stalks gotten rid of.

2 table spoon granulated sugar.

300ml water.

Action.

Set up the raspberries in 2 serving dishes/glasses/moulds. Location the gelatine leaves in a bowl of cold water to soften.

Place the blackcurrants in a small pan with the sugar and 100ml water and give the boil. Simmer intensely for 5 minutes and after that remove from the very first heat. Delegate stand for 2 minutes.

Squeeze out excess water from the gelatine leaves and include them to the pan. Stir till completely liquified, then stir in the rest of the water. Pour the liquid into the prepared dishes and refrigerate to set. The jellies should be prepared in about 3-4 hours or overnight.

APPLE PANCAKES WITH BLACKCURRANT COMPOTE.

337 calories.

1 1/2 of you SIRT 5 a day.

These pancakes are healthy however decadent. A terrific lazy morning reward.

Dispense s 4 - Ready in 20 minutes.

Things required.

75g porridge oats.

125g plain flour.

1 tea spoon baking powder.

2 table spoon caster sugar.

Pinch of salt.

2 apples, peeled, cored and cut into little pieces.

300ml semi-skimmed milk.

2 egg whites.

2 tea spoon light olive oil.

For the compote:

120g blackcurrants, cleaned and stalks eliminated.

2 table spoon caster sugar.

3 table spoon water.

Action.

Make the compote. Place the blackcurrants, sugar, and water in a little pan. Bring up to a simmer and cook for 10-15 minutes.

Place the oats, flour, baking powder, caster sugar and salt in a big bowl and mix well. Stir in the apple and then blend in the milk a little at a time up until you have a smooth mixture. Whisk the egg whites to stiff peaks and then fold into the pancake batter. Transfer the batter to a container.

Very first heat 1/2 tea spoon oil in a non-stick frying pan on a medium-high first heat and gather roughly one quarter of the batter. Cook on both sides up until golden brown. Repeat and eliminate to make 4 pancakes.

Dispense the pancakes with the blackcurrant compote drizzled over.

SIRT FRUIT SALAD.

172 calories.

3 of your SIRT 5 a day.

This fruit salad is jam-packed full of the very best fruit SIRTs.

Dish out s 1 - Ready in 10 minutes.

Things needed.

1/2 cup freshly made green tea.

1 tea spoon honey.

1 orange, cut in half.

1 apple, cored and approximately sliced.

10 red seedless grapes.

10 blueberries.

Action.

Stir the honey into half a cup of green tea. When dissolved, include the juice of half the orange. Delegate cool.

Chop the other half of the orange and place in a bowl together with the sliced apple, blueberries and grapes. Pour over the cooled tea and leave to steep for a couple of minutes before serving.

SIRTFOOD BITES-SIRTFOOD RECIPES.

THINGS NEEDED.

120g walnuts.

30g dark chocolate (85 per cent cocoa solids), gotten into pieces; or cocoa nibs.

250g Medjool dates pitted.

1 table spoon cocoa powder.

1 table spoon ground turmeric.

1 table spoon additional virgin olive oil.

the scraped seeds of one vanilla pod or 1 teaspoon

vanilla extract.

1-- 2 table spoon water.

ACTIONS.

Location the walnuts and chocolate in a food processor and process up until you have a fine powder.

Consist of all the other things required other than the water and blend up until the mixture forms a ball. You might or might not need to consist of the water depending upon the consistency of the mixture-- you do not desire it to be too sticky.

Using your hands, form the mixture into bite-sized balls and refrigerate in an airtight container for a minimum of one hour before consuming them.

You could roll a few of the balls in some more cocoa or desiccated coconut to attain a various surface if you like.

They will keep for as much as one week in your fridge.

SIRT MUESLI-SIRTFOOD RECIPES.

Things needed:

20g buckwheat flakes.

10g buckwheat puffs.

15g coconut flakes or desiccated coconut.

40g Medjool dates, pitted and chopped.

15g walnuts, sliced.

10g cocoa nibs.

100g strawberries, hulled and chopped.

100g plain Greek yoghurt (or vegan option, such as soya or coconut yoghurt).

Steps:

Mix all of the above things needed together, just including the yogurt and strawberries before serving if you are making it wholesale.

CHINESE-STYLE PORK WITH PAK CHOI-SIRTFOOD RECIPES.

377 CALORIES AND 2 OF YOUR SIRT 5 A DAY.

Dispense s 4.

Things needed.

400g firm tofu, cut into large cubes.

1 table spoon cornflour.

1 table spoon water.

125ml chicken stock.

1 table spoon rice white wine.

1 table spoon tomato purée.

1 tea spoon brown sugar.

1 table spoon soy sauce.

1 clove garlic, peeled and squashed.

1 thumb (5cm) fresh ginger, peeled and grated 1 table spoon rapeseed oil.

100g shiitake mushrooms, sliced.

1 shallot, peeled and sliced.

200g pak choi or choi amount, cut into thin slices
400g pork mince (10% fat).

100g beansprouts.

Large handful (20g) parsley, sliced.

Here's how:

Lay out the tofu on kitchen area paper, cover with more kitchen area paper and reserved.

In a small bowl, mix together the cornflour and water, getting rid of all lumps. Include the chicken stock, rice wine, tomato purée, brown sugar and soy sauce. Consist of the crushed garlic and ginger and stir together.

Eliminate the mushrooms from the pan with a slotted spoon and set aside. Eliminate with a slotted spoon and set aside.

Include the shallot and pak choi to the wok, stir-fry for 2 minutes, then include the mince. Prepare till the mince is prepared through, then include the sauce, minimize the first heat a notch and enable the sauce to bubble round the meat for a minute or 2. Include the beansprouts, shiitake mushrooms and tofu to the pan and warm through. Remove from the very first heat, stir through the parsley and dish out immediately.

TUSCAN BEAN STEW.

Things needed.

1 table spoon additional virgin olive oil.

50g red onion, finely sliced.

30g carrot, peeled and carefully sliced.

30g celery, trimmed and carefully sliced.

1 garlic clove, carefully sliced.

1/2 bird's eye chili, finely sliced (optional).

1 tea spoon herbes de Provence.

200ml veggie stock.

1 x 400g tin sliced Italian tomatoes.

1 tea spoon tomato purée.

200g tinned combined beans.

50g kale, approximately chopped.

1 table spoon roughly sliced parsley.

40g buckwheat.

Method. Place the oil in a medium pan over a low--medium first heat and carefully fry the onion, carrot, celery, garlic, chilli(if utilizing) and herbs, till the onion is soft but not colored.

Include the stock, tomatoes and tomato purée and bring to the boil. Consist of the beans and simmer for 30 minutes.

Include the kale and cook for another 5-- 10 minutes, till tender, then consist of the parsley.

Cook the buckwheat according to the package steps, drain and then dish out with the stew.

SALMON SIRT SUPER SALAD.

Makes 1.

Things required.

50g rocket.

50g chicory leaves.

100g smoked salmon slices (you can also use lentils, cooked chicken breast or tinned tuna).

80g avocado, peeled, stoned and sliced.

40g celery, sliced.

20g red onion, sliced.

15g walnuts, sliced.

1 tbs caper.

1 large Medjool date, pitted and chopped.

1 tbs extra-virgin olive oil.

Juice 1/4 lemon.

10g parsley, sliced.

10g lovage or celery leaves, chopped.

Steps.

Arrange the salad leaves on a big plate. Mix all the staying things required together and dish out on top of the leaves.

Turkey Escalope with sage, parsley and caper and spiced cauliflower 'couscous'.

* 150g cauliflower, approximately sliced.

* 1 clove garlic, finely sliced.

* 40g red onion, finely chopped.

* 1 bird's eye chilli, finely chopped.

* 1tea spoon fresh ginger, carefully chopped.

* 2table spoon additional virgin olive oil.

* 2tea spoon ground turmeric.

* 30g sun-dried tomatoes, carefully chopped.

* 10g parsley.

* 150g turkey escalope.

* 1tea spoon dried sage.

* Juice 1/2 lemon.

* 1table spoon capers.

Place the cauliflower in a food processor and pulse in 2-second bursts to carefully chop it up until it looks like couscous. Set aside. Fry the garlic, red onion, chilli and ginger in 1tea spoon of the oil till soft but not coloured. Consist of the turmeric and cauliflower and cook for 1 minute. Get rid of from the first heat and consist of the sun-dried tomatoes and half the parsley.

Cover the turkey escalope in the staying oil and sage then fry for 5-6 minutes, turning routinely. When cooked, include the lemon juice, remaining parsley, capers and 1table spoon water to the pan to make a sauce, then dispense.

SIRTFOOD DIET'S BRAISED PUY LENTILS.

Dish outs: 1.

Preparation time: 40-- 50 minutes.

Things required.

8 Cherry tomatoes, cut in half.

2 tea spoon Extra virgin olive oil.

40 g Red onion, very finely sliced.

1 Garlic clove, carefully chopped.

40 g Celery, thinly sliced.

40 g Carrots, peeled and very finely sliced.

1 tea spoon Paprika.

1 tea spoon Thyme (fresh or dry).

75 g Puy lentils.

220 ml Vegetable stock.

50 g Kale, approximately sliced.

1 table spoon Parsley, sliced.

20 g Rocket.

Approach.

1. Place the tomatoes into a little roasting tin and roast in the microwave oven for 35-- 45 minutes.

3. Heat a saucepan over a low-- medium first heat. Consist of 1 teaspoon of the olive oil with the red onion, celery, carrot, and garlic and fry for 1-- 2 minutes, until softened. Stir in the paprika and thyme and cook for an additional minute.

4. Wash the lentils in a fine-meshed sieve and include them to the pan together with the stock. Give the boil, then reduce the very first heat and simmer carefully for 20 minutes with a lid on the pan. Offer the pan a stir every 7 minutes or two, including a little water if the level drops too much.

Include the kale and cook for a more 10 minutes. Dish out with the rocket sprinkled with the remaining teaspoon of olive oil.

SIRTFOOD DIET'S SHAKSHUKA.

Enjoy this healthy recipe of spicy baked eggs and kale.

Dispense s: 1.

Preparation time: 40 minutes.

Things required.

1 tea spoon Extra virgin olive oil.

40g Red onion, carefully chopped.

1 Garlic clove, finely chopped.

30g Celery, finely sliced.

1 Bird's eye chilli, finely chopped.

1 tea spoon Ground cumin.

1 tea spoon Ground turmeric.

1 teaspoon Paprika.

400g Tinned sliced tomatoes.

30g Kale, stems eliminated and roughly chopped.

1 tablespoon Chopped parsley.

2 Medium eggs.

Approach.

1. Heat a small, deep-sided frying pan over a medium-- low first heat. Consist of the oil and fry the onion, garlic, celery, chilli and spices for 1-- 2 minutes.

2. Include the tomatoes, then leave the sauce to simmer gently for 20 minutes, stirring periodically.

Include the kale and cook for a further 5 minutes. If you feel the sauce is getting too thick, simply consist of a little water.

Decrease the very first heat to its most affordable setting and cover the pan with a cover or foil. Leave the eggs to cook for 10-- 12 minutes, at which point the whites should be firm while the yolks are still runny. Prepare for a more 3-- 4 minutes if you choose the yolks to be firm.

VIETNAMESE TURMERIC FISH WITH HERBS & MANGO SAUCE-NEW.

Prep time: 15 minutes Cook time 30 mins Total 45 minutes.

Things needed.

Fish:

* 1 1/4 pounds fresh cod boneless, skinless and fish, cut into 2-inch piece large that have to do with 1/2 inch thick.

If essential), * 2 table spoon coconut oil to pan-fry the fish (plus a couple of more tablespoon.

* Small pinch of sea salt to taste.

Fish marinade: (Marinate for at least 1 hr. or as long as overnight).

* 1 table spoon turmeric powder.

* 1 teaspoon sea salt.

* 1 table spoon Chinese cooking red wine (Alt. dry sherry).

* 2 tea spoon minced ginger.

* 2 table spoon olive oil.

Instilled Scallion and Dill Oil:.

* 2 cups scallions (piece into long thin shape).

* 2 cups of fresh dill.

* Pinch of sea salt to taste.

Mango dipping sauce:

* 1 medium sized ripe mango.

* 2 table spoon rice vinegar.

* Juice of 1/2 lime.

1 garlic clove.

1 tea spoon dry red chili pepper (stir in prior to serving).

Toppings:

* Fresh cilantro (as much as you like).

* Lime juice (as much as you like).

* Nuts (cashew or pine nuts).

Steps.

Actions:

1. Marinade the fish for a minimum of 1 hr. or as long as over night.

2. Location all things required under "Mango Dipping Sauce" into a food mill and blend till wanted consistency.

To Pan-Fry The Fish:

First heat 2 table spoon of coconut oil in a non-stick big frying pan over high very first heat. When hot, consist of the pre-marinated fish. * Note: place the fish slices into the pan individually and separate to two or more batches to pan fry if essential.

You should hear a loud sizzle, after which you can reduce the very first heat to medium-high.

Do not move the fish or turn up until you see a golden brown color on the side, about 5 minutes. Season with a pinch of sea salt. Consist of of more coconut oil to pan-fry the fish is essential.

* Note: There need to be some oil left in the frying pan. We utilize the remainder of the oil to make scallion and dill instilled oil.

To Make The Scallion And Dill Infused Oil:.

Utilize the rest of the oil in the fry pan over medium-high first heat, include 2 cups of scallions and 2 cups of dill. Once you have actually includeed the scallions and dill, turn off the first heat. Provide a gentle toss just up until the scallions and dill have actually wilted, about 15 seconds. Season with a dash of sea salt.

Pour the scallion, dill, and instilled oil over the fish and dish outwith mango dipping sauce with fresh cilantro, lime, and nuts.

MOROCCAN SPICED EGGS.

394 calories.

MEAL OUT S 2 - READY IN 50 MINUTES.

Things needed.

1 tea spoon olive oil.

1 shallot, peeled and finely chopped.

1 red (bell) pepper, deseeded and finely sliced.

1 garlic clove, peeled and carefully chopped.

1 courgette (zucchini), peeled and finely chopped.

1 table spoon tomato puree (paste).

1/2 tea spoon mild chilli powder.

1/4 tea spoon ground cinnamon.

1/4 tea spoon ground cumin.

1/2 tea spoon salt.

1 × 400g (14oz) can sliced tomatoes.

1 x 400g (14oz) can chickpeas in water.

small handful of flat-leaf parsley (10g (1/3oz)), sliced.

4 medium eggs at room temperature.

Action.

- First heat the oil in a saucepan, include the shallot and red (bell) pepper and fry carefully for 5 minutes. Include the garlic and courgette (zucchini) and cook for another minute or two. Consist of the tomato puree (paste), spices and salt and stir through.

- Include the chopped tomatoes and chickpeas (soaking alcohol and all) and increase the very first heat to medium. With the cover off the pan, simmer the sauce for 30 minutes-- make sure it is gently bubbling throughout and permit it to minimize in volume by about one-third.

- Remove from the very first heat and stir in the chopped parsley.

- Prefirst heat the microwave oven to 200C/180C fan/350F.

- When you are prepared to cook the eggs, bring the tomato sauce as much as a gentle simmer and transfer to a little microwave oven-proof meal.

- Crack the eggs on the side of the meal and lower them gently into the stew. Cover with foil and bake in the microwave oven for 10-15 minutes. Meal outthe concoction in individual bowls with the eggs drifting on the top.

RAW BROWNIE BITES.

Overall Time: 5 minutes.

Dispense s: 6.

THINGS NEEDED:

2 1/2 cups entire walnuts.

1/4 cup almonds.

2 1/2 cups Medjool dates.

1 cup cacao powder.

1 teaspoon vanilla extract.

⅛- 1/4 teaspoon sea salt.

STEPS:

Location everything in a food mill till well

integrated.

Roll into balls and put on a baking sheet and freeze for 30 minutes or refrigerate for 2 hours.

WALDORF SALAD.

Things needed (meal out s 2).

200g celery, approximately chopped.

100g apple, approximately sliced.

50g walnuts, roughly sliced.

1 little red onion, approximately sliced.

1 head of chicory, chopped.

10g flat parsley, sliced.

1 tablespoon capers.

10g lovage or celery leaves, approximately chopped.

For the dressing:

1 table spoon extra virgin olive oil.

1 teaspoon balsamic vinegar.

1 teaspoon Dijon mustard.

Juice of half a lemon.

Action.

Mix the celery, apple, walnuts, onion, parsley, capers and lovage/celery in a medium-sized salad bowl and mix. Make the dressing by whisking together the.

oil, vinegar, mustard and lemon juice.Drizzle over the salad, mix and dish out!

FRESH SAAG PANEER.

279 calories.

3 of your SIRT 5 a day.

Dish out s 2 - Ready in 20 minutes.

Things needed.

2 tea spoon rapeseed oil.

200g paneer. cut into cubes.

Salt and newly ground black pepper.

1 red onion, sliced.

1 small thumb (3 cm) fresh ginger, peeled and cut into matchsticks.

1 clove garlic, peeled and thinly sliced.

1 green chilli, deseeded and finely sliced.

100g cherry tomatoes, cut in half.

1/2 tea spoon ground coriander.

1/2 tea spoon ground cumin.

1/4 tea spoon ground turmeric.

1/2 tea spoon moderate chilli powder.

1/2 tea spoon salt.

100g fresh spinach leaves.

Little handful (10g) parsley, chopped.

Little handful (10g) coriander, chopped.

Steps.

Fry for a few minutes until golden, stirring frequently. Remove from the pan with a slotted spoon and set aside.

Reduce the first heat and include the onion. Fry for 5 minutes before including the garlic, chilli and ginger. Cook for another couple of minutes prior to including the cherry tomatoes. Place the lid on the pan and cook for an additional 5 minutes.

Include the spices and salt, then stir. Return the paneer to the pan and stir up until layered. Consist of the spinach to the pan together with the parsley and coriander and place the lid on. Enable the spinach to wilt for 1-2 minutes, then include into the meal. Dish out immediately.

SWEET POTATO AND SALMON PATTIES.

Things needed.

225g/8oz wild salmon, cooked or tinned.

225g/8oz sweet potato mashed and prepared.

Herb salt and pepper to taste.

Rice flour or buckwheat flour.

Action.

Prefirst heat the microwave to 160C/gas mark 3.

Mix together the sweet potato, salmon, herb salt and pepper. Take a small handful of the mixture and roll into a ball shape. Flatten into a hamburger shape then dip each side in the flour. Put on a lined baking tray. Repeat up until you have utilized up the mixture.

Bake for 20 minutes turning once. Dish outwith a big green salad.

MOONG DAHL.

Dish out s 4-6.

Things needed.

300g/10oz split mung beans (moong dahl)-- preferably soaked for a couple of hours.

600ml/1pt of water.

2 table spoon/30g olive butter, oil or ghee.

1 red onion, finely chopped.

1-2 tea spoon coriander seeds.

1-2 tea spoon cumin seeds.

2-4 tea spoon fresh ginger, sliced.

1-2 tea spoon turmeric.

If you desire it spicy, 1/4 tea spoon of cayenne

pepper-- more.

Salt & black pepper to taste.

Action.

Drain and wash the split mung beans. Put them in a pan and cover with the water. Give the boil and skim off any foam that occurs. Decline the very first heat, cover and simmer.

First heat the oil in a pan and sauté the onion till soft.

Dry fry the coriander and cumin seeds in a heavy bottomed pan up until they start to pop. Grind them in a pestle and mortar.

Consist of the ground spices to the onions in addition to the cayenne, turmeric and ginger pepper. Cook for a few minutes.

When the mung beans are almost cooked include the onion and spice mix to them. Season with salt and pepper and cook for an additional 10 minutes.

DILL ROASTED MACKEREL WITH TOMATOES AND STEAMED VEGETABLES

Dish outs 2

Things required

Olive oil

A handful of dill fronds

2 mackerel fillets

1 beef tomato, finely sliced

Salt and pepper

Vegetables for steaming; eg; kale, carrots, chard

Juice of one lemon.

Action

Prefirst heat the microwave oven to 220C/gas mark 7

Brush a microwave oven evidence dish with olive oil and spread the dill leaves on top. Place the fish on top of this and top with the sliced tomato. Season with salt and pepper.

Cover with foil and bake for 10-15 minutes until the fish is prepared through.

Steam the vegetables for 5-10 minutes and dispense with the fish. Squeeze the lemon juice over the fish and veggies.

BUCKWHEAT BEAN AND TOMATO RISOTTO

Dispense s 4

Things required

2 table spoon olive oil or butter

2 cloves of garlic, chopped

225g/8oz buckwheat

400ml of hot water or vegetable stock

225g/8oz frozen broad beans

1/2 cup of sun-dried tomatoes in oil

Juice of half a lemon

2 table spoon basil or coriander, sliced

50g/2oz almonds, toasted

Salt and pepper

Step

Heat the olive oil or butter in a frying pan. Consist of the garlic and cook for a minute.

Consist of the buckwheat to the pan and stir it well to coat it in the oil.

Consist of the hot water or stock. Cover and simmer for 10 minutes.

Stir in the broad beans. Cook for a few minutes till the beans are just tender.

Include the sun-dried tomatoes, lemon juice, fresh herbs and almonds and season with salt and pepper.

TROUT WITH ROASTED VEGETABLES

Dish out s 2

Things required

2 carrots, cut into batons

2 parsnips, peeled and cut into wedges

2 turnips, peeled and cut into sections

Olive oil

Juice of 1 lemon

Tamari

1 trout fillet per person

Dried dill

Step

Location the sliced vegetables on a baking tray. Sprinkle with olive oil and a dash of tamari. Place in the microwave oven on gas mark 7. After 25 minutes, take the veggies out of the microwave oven and stir them well.

Place the fish on top of them. Sprinkle with lemon juice and dill. Cover with foil and go back to the microwave.

Turn the microwave to gas mark 5/190C/375F and cook for 20 minutes up until the fish is prepared through.

COURGETTE TORTILLA

Dispense s 2

Things required

2 table spoon coconut oil or butter

1 courgettes, sliced

4 eggs, beaten

A pinch of salt and pepper

Newly chopped chives or parsley

Action

First heat the oil or butter in a heavy bottomed fry pan and consist of the courgettes. Prepare until soft, stirring sometimes.

Mix the salt, pepper, and herbs in with the beaten eggs and consist of to the pan

Cook till the egg is almost cooked through. End up the cooking by positioning the pan under a medium grill. Dish out with a large green salad.

POLENTA BAKE

Dish out s 4-6

Things needed

850ml/1.5 pints of water

1 tea spoon rock salt or sea salt

200g/7oz coarse yellow polenta

2 tea spoon dried oregano

1 cup of sun-dried tomatoes, sliced

3 eggs, separated

1-2 table spoon butter or olive oil

Freshly ground black pepper

300g/10oz cheddar or red Leicester cheese, grated (optional).

Step.

To cook the polenta bring the water to the boil in a large pan with the salt.

Gradually gather the polenta stirring all the time. Consist of the oregano and the sun-dried tomatoes.

Prepare on a low very first heat for as long as the actions on the polenta packet indicate. It might be anywhere from 3 minutes to 40 minutes. Stir routinely to prevent clumping and sticking.

While the polenta is cooking whip the egg whites until they form stiff peaks.

As soon as the polenta is cooked shut off the first

heat and stir in 1-2 table spoon of butter or olive oil along with 2/3 of the cheese (if using), the egg yolks and black pepper. If needed, include more salt.

Fold the egg whites thoroughly into the polenta mix.

Transfer the mix to an oiled microwave evidence meal. Spread out and smooth the top.

Spray on the rest of the grated cheese.

Bake at gas mark 4/180C/350F for 40-50 minutes until set and beginning to brown.

BUTTERBEAN AND VEGETABLE KORMA.

Dispense s 4.

Things needed.

3 tablespoon coconut oil or olive oil.

1 big onion, carefully sliced.

2 tea spoon root ginger, finely sliced.

1 clove of garlic, finely chopped.

1-2 table spoon curry powder.

200g/7oz green beans, cut into 2 cm lengths.

1 cauliflower, cut into florets.

3 sweet potatoes, peeled and sliced into large pieces.

2 cans of butterbeans (or prepare your own utilizing 225g/8oz of dried beans).

50-100g/ 2-4oz creamed coconut.

1 table spoon sliced coriander.

Step.

First heat the oil in a large saucepan and consist of the onion. Cook up until the onions are soft.

Include the ginger and garlic, to the onions and cook for a couple of more minutes.

Stir in the curry powder then consist of the green beans, cauliflower and sweet potatoes and stir well to coat them in the spices.

Consist of the drained pipes and rinsed butterbeans and sufficient hot water to simply cover the important things required.

Prepare for 20-30 minutes or until the vegetables are prepared through.

Transfer a few of the liquid from the pan into bowl and dissolve the creamed coconut in it. Include this to the pan and cook for a few minutes.

Spray on the fresh coriander just prior to serving.

BAKED SALMON WITH STIR-FRIED VEGETABLES.

Dish out s 2.

Things required.

Grated zest and juice of 1 lemon.

2 teaspoon of root ginger, grated.

2 wild salmon fillets.

1 tea spoon toasted sesame oil.

2 teaspoon olive oil.

2 carrots, cut into matchsticks.

Lot of kale, sliced.

1 tin of water chestnuts, drained pipes, rinsed and chopped.

Action.

Mix together lemon juice and zest and ginger. Place the salmon in a shallow, microwave evidence dish and pour over the ginger lemon mixture. Cover with foil and leave to marinade for 30-60 minutes.

Bake the salmon in the microwave for 15 minutes on gas mark 5/190C.

While it is cooking very first heat a wok or frying pan and include the toasted sesame oil and olive oil. Include the veggies and cook for a couple of minutes, stirring continuously.

When the salmon is cooked spoon some of the marinade from the salmon onto the veggies and cook for a couple more minutes.

Meal outthe veggies onto a plate and place the salmon on top.

LEMON PAPRIKA CHICKEN WITH VEGETABLES.

Dispense s 2.

Things required.

3 tablespoon olive oil.

2 table spoon paprika.

2 carrots, chopped.

1/2 a celeriac, peeled and chopped.

3 turnips, peeled and sliced.

300g of chicken wings.

1 pint of hot stock.

Sprigs of rosemary and thyme.

2 bay leaves.

Salt and pepper.

Juice of 1 lemon.

Large lot of kale, chopped.

Action.

Very first heat the oil in a large pan with a tight fitting cover. Include the paprika, carrots, celeriac, chicken and turnip wings to the pan and cook for a couple of minutes.

Consist of the stock, herbs, salt, pepper and lemon juice to the pan and give the boil.

Turn down the very first heat, cover with a lid and simmer carefully for 40 minutes.

Consist of the kale and cook for a couple of more minutes until the kale and chicken are both cooked.

RAW CARROT AND ALMOND LOAF.

Things needed.

6-8 carrots, grated.

Juice of 1/2 a lemon.

1/2 cup of almonds.

Fresh parsley, finely sliced.

4 table spoon of tahini.

Action.

Location the grated carrots into a food processor with the S blade.

Whizz the carrots up with the lemon juice till they are well homogenized. Put them in a bowl.

Then whizz up the almonds in the food processor until they are ground down.

Include the carrot mix to the almonds and blend them all together with the sliced parsley and tahini.

Pack this into a loaf tin and cut into pieces to dispense.

Savory SEED TRUFFLES.

Things required.

60g/2oz pumpkin seeds.

60g/2oz sunflower seeds.

2 table spoon tahini.

Pinch of cayenne pepper.

Juice of half a lemon.

A handful of coriander leaves.

Salt and pepper.

Step.

Place the seeds in a food mill with the S blade and grind thoroughly.

Include the tahini, cayenne, lemon juice, coriander leaves and salt and pepper.

Process till the mix holds together includeing little quantities of water as required.

Get rid of the blade from the food mill and form the mix into walnut sized balls.

ALMOND BUTTER AND ALFALFA WRAPS.

Things required.

4 tablespoon of almond nut butter.

Juice of 1 lemon.

2-3 carrots-- grated.

3 radishes, carefully sliced.

1 cup of alfalfa sprouts.

Salt and pepper.

Lettuce leaves or nori sheets.

Step.

Mix the almond butter with the majority of the lemon juice and enough water to create a velvety consistency.

Combine the grated carrot, alfalfa sprouts in a bowl. Sprinkle with the remainder of the lemon juice and season with salt and pepper.

Spread the lettuce leaves or nori sheets with almond butter and top with the carrot and grow mixture. Roll up and consume instantly!

BUCKWHEAT PANCAKES.

Dispense s 4.

Things needed.

110g/4oz buckwheat flour.

1/2 tea spoon of salt.

1 free range egg, beaten.

1 cup of natural soya yoghurt (or other natural yoghurt).

1 cup of water.

Butter, olive oil or coconut oil for frying.

Step.

Combine the flour and salt in a blending bowl and make a well in the centre.

Combine the egg, yoghurt and water in container and slowly beat this into the flour up until you have a smooth batter. Leave to rest for an hour or more.

Heat some oil in a frying pan and drop tablespoons of the batter into the pan.

Cook for a few minutes up until the underside is starting to brown before gently turning over. Cook for a couple more minutes up until cooked.

Continue till you have utilized all the batter.

PEA, MISO, AND MINT SOUP.

Things required.

2 table spoon olive oil.

1 red onion (optional), carefully sliced.

300g/10oz of frozen peas.

2 table spoon fresh mint, sliced.

1 tea spoon miso.

Salt and pepper.

4 table spoon natural yoghurt or soya yoghurt (optional).

Step.

Heat the oil in a pan and consist of the onion.

Prepare till they are soft.

Include the frozen peas and 700ml of boiling water.

Give the boil and simmer for a couple of minutes.

Include the mint, salt, pepper and miso and mix with a hand blender till smooth.

Meal out into bowls and swirl in the yoghurt if utilizing.

BUCKWHEAT NOODLE AND GREEN BEAN SOUP.

Dispense s 4.

Things required.

2 table spoon olive oil.

1 tea spoon toasted sesame oil.

1 tea spoon ginger root, finely sliced.

2 spring onions, finely sliced.

2 carrots, cut into thin strips.

1 litre of boiling water.

400g buckwheat noodles.

1 table spoon tamari soy sauce.

1 table spoon rice white wine (optional).

125g/4oz frozen edamame beans.

Fresh coriander, finely chopped.

Salt and pepper.

Action.

Heat the olive and sesame oil in a wok or large saucepan. Stir in the ginger root, spring onions, and carrots and cook for a couple of minutes.

Put in a litre of boiling water. Once it is bubbling consist of the noodles, tamari, rice red wine and edamame beans.

Prepare until the vegetables and noodles are just cooked.

If desired, garnish with coriander leaves and season with salt and pepper.

AVOCADO AND CANNELLINI MASH TACOS.

Dispense s 2.

Things needed.

1 ripe avocado, peeled and stoned.

1 400g can of cannellini beans, drained.

Juice of 1/2 a lemon.

1 table spoon olive oil.

Salt and pepper.

A couple of basil leaves.

Taco shells.

Step.

Place the avocado into a bowl, approximately chop it and then mash it.

Consist of the cannellini beans and lemon juice and mash them all together.

Stir in the olive oil and season with salt and pepper. Destroy the basil leaves and consist of these.

Fill the taco shells and consume instantly!

GREEN BEAN, TOMATO, AND ALMOND STIR FRY.

Dish outs 4.

Things needed.

2 table spoon olive oil.

1 tea spoon root ginger, finely sliced.

1 clove of garlic, finely chopped.

450g/1lb of green beans eg: Runner beans, French beans, and Sugar Snap Peas sliced into 2cm lengths.

Passion and juice of half a lemon.

1 table spoon of tamari.

A dash of toasted sesame oil.

2 tomatoes, sliced.

2 table spoon almonds, toasted.

Salt and pepper.

A handful of basil leaves.

Step.

First heat the oil in a pan include the root ginger

and cook for a couple of minutes. Include the garlic and cook for a minute.

Consist of the sliced beans, lemon juice, a dash of toasted sesame oil, a dash of tamari and a couple of tablespoons of water. Cover the pan with a cover and cook for 5-10 minutes until the beans are simply prepared. If it begins to dry out, consist of more water after a couple of minutes.

Stir in the tomatoes, almonds and lemon passion, season with salt and pepper, sprinkle on the basil leaves and dish out right away.

MOCHA CHOCOLATE MOUSSE-NEW SIRTFOOD RECIPES.

Everyone takes pleasure in chocolate mousse and this one has a wonderful light and airy texture. It is simple and quick to make and is best dispense d the day after it's made.

Dish out s 4-- 6.

Things required.

250g dark chocolate (85% cocoa solids).

6 medium free-range eggs, separated.

4 table spoon strong black coffee.

4 table spoon almond milk.

Chocolate coffee beans, to embellish.

Steps:

Melt the chocolate in a big bowl set over a pan of gently simmering water, ensuring the bottom of the bowl does not touch the water. Eliminate the bowl from the first heat and leave the melted chocolate to cool to space temperature level.

When the melted chocolate is at space temperature, whisk in the egg yolks one at a time and then carefully fold in the coffee and almond milk.

Using a hand-held electric mixer, blend the egg whites up until stiff peaks form, then blend a couple of tablespoons into the chocolate mixture to loosen it. Carefully fold in the rest, using a big metal spoon.

Transfer the mousse to individual glasses and smooth the surface area. Cover with stick film and chill for a minimum of 2 hours, ideally overnight. Decorate with chocolate coffee beans prior to serving.

BUCKWHEAT PANCAKES WITH STRAWBERRIES, DARK CHOCOLATE SAUCE AND CRUSHED WALNUTS

Makes around 6 to 8 pancakes, depending on the size.

For the pancakes you will need:

350ml milk

150g buckwheat flour

1 big egg

1 table spoon additional virgin olive oil, for cooking

For the chocolate sauce

100g dark chocolate (85 percent cocoa solids).

85ml milk.

1 table spoon double cream.

1 table spoon additional virgin olive oil.

To dispense.

400g strawberries, hulled and sliced.

100g walnuts, chopped.

Step.

To make the pancake batter, location all of the things needed apart from the olive oil in a blender and blend up until you have a smooth batter. (You can store any excess batter in an airtight container for up to 5 days in your refrigerator.

To make the chocolate sauce, melt the chocolate in a very first heatproof bowl over a pan of simmering water. As soon as melted, mix in the milk, whisking thoroughly and then consist of the double cream and olive oil. You can keep the sauce warm by leaving the water in the pan simmering on a very low very first heat until your pancakes are all set.

To make the pancakes very first heat a heavy-bottomed fry pan till it starts to smoke, then consist of the olive oil.

Pour a few of the batter into the centre of the pan, then tip the excess batter around it until you have actually covered the entire surface area, you may have to consist of a little bit more batter to achieve this. If your pan is hot enough, you will just need to cook the pancake for 1 minute or so on each side.

Once you can see it going brown around the edges utilize a spatula to loosen the pancake around its edge, then turn it over. Attempt to flip in one action to prevent breaking it.

Cook for an additional minute or two on the other side and transfer to a plate.

Place some strawberries in the centre and roll up the pancake. Continue till you have actually made as lots of pancakes as required.

Spoon over a generous amount of sauce and spray over some chopped walnuts.

You might discover that your very first efforts are too fat or break down but once you discover the consistency of your batter that works best for you and you get your strategy refined you'll be making them like an expert. Practice makes perfect in this case.

BLUEBERRY BANANA PANCAKES WITH CHUNKY APPLE COMPOTE AND GOLDEN TUMERIC LATTE.

Things required.

For the Blueberry Banana Pancakes.

6 bananas.

6 eggs.

150g rolled oats.

2 tea spoon baking powder.

1/4 teaspoon salt.

25g blueberries.

For the Chunky Apple Compote.

2 apples.

5 dates (pitted).

1 tablespoon lemon juice.

1/4 teaspoon cinnamon powder.

pinch salt.

For the Golden Turmeric Latte.

3 cups coconut milk.

1 teaspoon turmeric powder.

1 teaspoon cinnamon powder.

1 teaspoon raw honey.

Pinch of black pepper (boosts absorption).

Tiny piece of fresh, peeled ginger root.

Pinch of cayenne pepper (optional).

Actions.

For the Blueberry Banana Pancakes.

Pop the rolled oats in a high-speed blender and pulse for 1 minute or up until an oat flour has actually formed. Tip: make sure your blender is really dry before doing this otherwise whatever will end up being soaked!

Now include the bananas, eggs, baking powder and salt to the mixer and pulse for 2 minutes up until a smooth batter forms.

Transfer the mix to a big bowl and fold in the blueberries. Delegate rest for 10 minutes whilst the baking powder activates.

To make your pancakes, include a dollop of butter (this assists to make them crispy and really delicious!) to your frying pan on a medium-high first heat. Include a few spoons of the blueberry pancake mix and fry for till well golden on the bottom side. Toss the pancake to fry the opposite.

For the Chunky Apple Compote.

Core and rough slice your apples.

Pop everything in a food processor, together with 2 tablespoons of water and a pinch of salt. Pulse to form your chunky apple compote.

For the Golden Turmeric Latte.

Mix all things required in a high-speed blender until smooth.

Put into a small pan and first heat for 4 minutes over medium very first heat till hot however not boiling.

Take pleasure in!

BLUEBERRY SMOOTHIE.

160 calories.

1 of your SIRT 5 a day.

This yogurt smoothie has an abundant, creamy taste.

Dish out s 2 - Ready in 2 minutes.

Things needed.

1 ripe banana.

100g blueberries.

100g blackberries.

2 table spoon natural yogurt.

200ml milk.

Blend all the things required together until smooth.

Savory Turmeric Pancakes With Lemon Yogurt Sauce.

Dish out s: 8 pancakes.

Things needed.

For The Yogurt Sauce.

1 cup plain Greek yogurt.

1 garlic clove, minced.

1 to 2 tablespoons lemon juice (from 1 lemon), to taste.

1/4 teaspoon ground turmeric.

10 fresh mint leaves, minced.

2 teaspoons lemon passion (from 1 lemon).

For The Pancakes.

2 teaspoons ground turmeric.

1 1/2 teaspoons ground cumin.

1 teaspoon salt.

1 teaspoon ground coriander.

1/2 teaspoon garlic powder.

1/2 teaspoon newly ground black pepper.

1 head broccoli, cut into florets.

3 big eggs, lightly beaten.

2 tablespoons plain unsweetened almond milk.

1 cup almond flour.

4 teaspoons coconut oil.

Actions.

Make the yogurt sauce. Integrate the yogurt, garlic, lemon juice, turmeric, mint and enthusiasm in a bowl. Taste and season with more lemon juice, if needed. Set aside or refrigerate up until prepared to dispense.

Make the pancakes. In a little bowl, combine the

turmeric, cumin, salt, pepper, garlic and coriander.

Place the broccoli in a food processor, and pulse until the florets are broken up into little pieces. Transfer the broccoli to a large bowl and consist of the eggs, almond milk, and almond flour. Stir in the spice mix and integrate well.

Prepare the pancake up until small bubbles start to appear on the surface and the bottom is golden brown, 2 to 3 minutes. Flip over and cook the pancake for 2 to 3 minutes more.

5. Continue making the remaining 3 pancakes, using the staying oil and batter.

SIRT CHILLI CON CARNE.

Dish outs 4.

1 red onion, finely sliced.

3 garlic cloves, carefully sliced.

2 bird's eye chilies, finely chopped.

1 table spoon additional virgin olive oil.

1 table spoon ground cumin.

1 table spoon ground turmeric.

400g lean minced beef (5 percent fat).

150ml red white wine.

1 red pepper, cored, seeds eliminated and cut into bite-sized pieces.

2 x 400g tins chopped tomatoes.

1 table spoon tomato purée.

1 table spoon cocoa powder.

150g tinned kidney beans.

300ml beef stock.

5g coriander, chopped.

5g parsley, chopped.

160g buckwheat.

In a casserole, fry the onion, garlic and chilli in the oil over a medium very first heat for 2-3 minutes, then consist of the spices and cook for a minute.

Include the minced beef and brown over a high very first heat. Include the red white wine and enable it to bubble to reduce it by half.

Consist of the red pepper, tomatoes, tomato purée, cocoa, kidney beans and stock and delegate simmer for 1 hour.

You may need to include a little water to accomplish a thick, sticky consistency.

Prior to serving, stir in the sliced herbs.

On the other hand, cook the buckwheat according to the packet actions and dish out with the chilli.

CHICKPEA, QUINOA AND TURMERIC CURRY RECIPE.

Dispense s 6.

Things required.

500g new potatoes, cut in half.

3 garlic cloves, crushed.

3 teaspoons ground turmeric.

1 teaspoon ground coriander.

1 teaspoon chilli flakes or powder.

1 teaspoon ground ginger.

400g can of coconut milk.

1 table spoon tomato purée.

400g can of chopped tomatoes.

salt and pepper.

180g quinoa.

400g can of chickpeas, drained pipes and rinsed.

150g spinach.

actions.

Place the potatoes in a pan of cold water and bring to the boil, then let them cook for about 25 minutes up until you can quickly stick a knife through them. Drain them well.

Location the potatoes in a large pan and consist of the garlic, turmeric, coriander, chilli, ginger, coconut milk, tomato purée and tomatoes. Bring to the boil, season with salt and pepper, then include the quinoa with a mug of just-boiled water (300ml).

Minimize the first heat to a simmer, put the lid on and permit to cook. Over the next 30 minutes, stirring every 5 minutes or two to ensure nothing sticks to the bottom. (This is rather a long cooking time, but this is for how long quinoa takes to cook in all these things required, instead of simply in water.) Halfway through cooking, include the chickpeas. When there are simply 5 minutes left, include the spinach and stir it in until it wilts. As soon as the quinoa has cooked and is fluffy, not crispy, it's ready.

Consist of a sliced red chilli to the cooking curry at the exact same time as the other spices if you like a bit of very first heat.

THE SIRTFOOD DIET GREEN JUICE SALAD.

An alternative to the Sirtfood Green Juice, this salad includes all the very same things needed as the green juice plus 2 additional Sirtfoods: walnuts and olive oil. Delicious and very easy to make.

Dish Type Main Course, Salad.

Cuisine British.

Preparation Time 10 minutes.

Overall Time 10 minutes.

Dispense s 1.

 Things needed.

Juice of 1/2 lemon.

1 cm ginger grated.

Salt and pepper to taste.

1 tablespoon olive oil.

2 handfuls kale sliced.

1 handful rocket.

1 tablespoon parsley.

2 celery sticks sliced.

1/2 green apple sliced.

6 walnut halves.

Method.

Location the lemon juice, ginger, salt, pepper and olive oil in a jam jar and shake to integrate.

Place the kale in a large bowl and pour over the dressing. Massage the dressing into the kale for 1 minute.

Include all the other things required and mix together completely.

CHRISTMAS TURKEY TRAYBAKE.

Preparation Time 20 minutes.

Prepare Time 55 minutes.

Total Time 1 hour 15 minutes.

Dispense s 4 (with leftovers).

Things required.

Olive oil.

1 kg baking potatoes peeled and cut into 50g chunks.

Salt and pepper.

500 g parsnips peeled cut into batons.

500 g chantenay carrots left whole.

8 garlic cloves gently slammed, skins left on.

1 large red onion cut and peeled into 8 wedges.

10 cocktail sausages wrapped in bacon you can purchase these ready prepared.

8 turkey breast fillets every one approximately 100g.

8 sage leaves.

200 g sprouts.

Gravy and other sauces to dish out.

Steps.

Pre-first heat your microwave to 200C. Drizzle about 8 tablespoons of olive oil in the base of a very big roasting tin (roughly 40 x 33cm) and put the tray in the microwave to very first warm up.

Consist of a teaspoon of salt and cook over a medium-high first heat for 12 minutes. (Start timing as quickly as you turn on the very first heat, NOT from when the water reboils).

Peel the parsnips and cut into big batons. I usually cut my parsnips in half lengthways and then widthways and then cut the leading part in half again lengthways so I get 6 approximately even sized batons.

Carefully slam 8 garlic cloves and peel and cut a red onion into quarters. Slice your sprouts in half and get the sage and carrots out of the refrigerator and you are all prepared.

When the potatoes are done, drain them and after that tip them into the hot fat. Spread them out and include the parsnips and carrots. Spray over an excellent quantity of salt and pepper and after that baste everything with a little of the hot fat (take care not to burn yourself!).

Location the tray in the microwave oven and roast for 20 minutes.

After 20 minutes remove the tray and consist of the garlic cloves, red onion wedges, mixed drink sausages and sage leaves. Offer everything another excellent baste and return the roasting tray to the microwave. Roast for another 20 minutes.

After 20 minutes, season the turkey breast fillets then include them to the tray along with the halved sprouts. Provide whatever another great baste and after that place back in the microwave oven for 15 minutes. This would be a great time to make a container of gravy and any other sauces you wish to dispense with the traybake (e.g. bread sauce and/or cranberry sauce).

After the last 15 minutes, check the turkey is done (cut the largest fillet in half and check it is white and not pink) and dish out with your gravy and sauces.

BEEF BOURGUIGNON STEW.

Preparation Time 30 minutes.

Cook Time 3 hours.

Total Time 3 hours 30 minutes.

Dispense s 4.

Things required.

200 g streaky bacon diced (or lardons).

12 little shallots peeled and chopped in half.

If truly huge), 200 g chestnut mushrooms sliced in half (or quarters.

800 g diced stewing beef offered from supermarkets or ask your butcher.

2 tablespoons plain flour.

300 ml red white wine I used Cono Sur Bicicleta Pinot Noir.

500 ml beef stock from a cube is great, I used 2 Kallo natural beef stock cubes.

2-3 bay leaves.

Salt and pepper.

Mashed potatoes and green veggies to dispense or simply crusty bread!

Steps.

Pre-first heat the microwave to 140C.

Location a non-stick frying pan on a medium/high very first heat and wait a number of minutes for the pan to first heat up. Location the pieces of bacon into the dry pan and fry for 3-4 minutes until crispy and actually brown, stirring frequently. Suggestion the bacon into a big microwave ovenproof meal (it should be one that has a lid).

Place the pan back onto the first heat and consist of a drizzle of olive oil and the shallots and mushrooms. Cook for about 3 minutes, stirring frequently, until the shallots and mushrooms are a golden brown on both sides. Tip into the microwave ovenproof dish.

Place the pan back on the first heat and consist of half the beef. Fry for about 2 minutes on each side up until golden brown. Tip into the microwave ovenproof dish and repeat with the other half of the beef.

When the 2nd great deal of beef is brown, deny the very first heat low and spray over the 2 tablespoons of plain flour. Stir to integrate, then include the red wine. Bring to the boil, stirring, then tip into the microwave ovenproof meal.

Make a quick stock using 2 beef stock cubes and 500ml boiling water. Idea the hot stock into the microwave ovenproof dish and include the bay leaves. Include salt and pepper to taste, then stir the contents of the microwave ovenproof meal so whatever is nicely integrated. Put the cover on the meal and location it in the microwave oven for 3 hours.

Dispense with mashed potatoes and vegetables or crusty bread.

BEST BANANA BREAD EVER.

Dish Type Cake.

Food British.

Preparation Time 15 minutes.

Prepare Time 45 minutes.

Total Time 1 hour.

Dish out s 16.

Things needed.

150 g unsalted butter melted.

200 g self-raising flour I utilized brown.

1/2 teaspoon bicarbonate of soda.

1/2 teaspoon salt.

150 g light soft brown sugar or caster sugar.

2 large eggs.

4 ripe bananas mashed.

50 g combined seeds or nuts optional.

Method.

Prefirst heat your microwave oven to 160C.

Place the butter in a little saucepan and melt carefully on a low very first heat. When all the butter is melted. Turn off and leave to cool for a few minutes.

Line 2 little (1lb) loaf tins with greaseproof paper. Scrunch up a sheet of greaseproof paper big enough to fit in one of your loaf tins. Wet it under the cold tap then utilize it to line the loaf tin. Repeat with the other tin.

Next, tip the flour into a big bowl and include the bicarbonate of salt, soda and sugar. Stir to integrate.

Peel the bananas and rip them into pieces. Location the banana chunks in a small bowl or container. Utilize a potato masher to mash them approximately then include the eggs and stir to combine.

Idea the eggs and banana mix into the dry things required and stir completely up until you have a thick batter. Consist of the cooled melted butter and stir well.

Consist of the nuts or seeds, if you are utilizing them, and stir as soon as more till the seeds are uniformly dispersed.

Divide the mix between the 2 loaf tins and cook the banana bread in your prefirst heated microwave oven for 45 minutes. If not prepare your banana bread for a more 5 minutes and examine again.

When your banana bread is prepared. Eliminate from the microwave oven. Allow to cool for 5 minutes then remove from the tin, peel off the greaseproof paper and cool on a cake rack ... or enjoy while it is still warm!

HOMEMADE CHICKEN FAJITAS.

These Homemade Chicken Fajitas are healthy, incredibly yummy and actually no less simple than their meal package cousins.

Dish Type Main Course.

Cuisine American, Mexican, Tex-Mex.

Preparation Time 5 minutes.

Prepare Time 10 minutes.

Overall Time 15 minutes.

Dish out s 4.

Things required.

12 flour or corn tortilla wraps I use Old El Paso.

2 teaspoons cumin.

If you like things hot, 1 teaspoon cayenne pepper more!

2 teaspoons dried oregano.

Juice of 1 lime.

2 cloves garlic grated or squashed.

2 large chicken breasts sliced into thin strips.

2 large onions sliced.

3 peppers I like to utilize a mix of colours, sliced into strips.

Olive oil.

2 tablespoons fresh coriander sliced finely.

Your choice of guacamole/ sour cream/ salsa/ grated cheese/ extra limes & coriander/ tortilla chips to dish out- any or all of them!

Approach.

If you are making your own guacamole or salsa, make these first and refrigerate till required-- or ask somebody else to make these for you while you get on with the fajitas.

Prefirst heat your microwave oven to 200C.

Get rid of the tortilla wraps from the package and wrap in foil.

Mix together the cumin, cayenne pepper, oregano, lime juice and crushed garlic in a large bowl.

Slice the chicken into thin strips and location in the marinade. Toss the chicken to thoroughly coat in the marinade and set aside for 5 minutes (or location in the refrigerator and marinade for longer if you prefer).

Utilize the time while the chicken is marinating to slice the peppers and onions.

When the microwave oven has actually initially warmed up, position the tortilla wraps in the microwave oven for 8 minutes up until warmed through. After 8 minutes eliminate from the microwave however keep covered in foil till required.

Fry the onions and peppers in a little olive oil on a low very first heat for 5 minutes until not brown but softened. Turn up the first heat and consist of the chicken and marinade and fry for about 5 minutes until the chicken is prepared through and browned and the veg is a little charred.

To inspect if the chicken is prepared all the way through, pick the thickest piece of chicken and cut it in half-- if it is totally white with no pink, it is cooked. And if the thickest piece is cooked, so ought to all the slimmers ones!

Spray the chicken with the chopped coriander and meal out in the pan on the table, together with the warm tortilla wraps and whatever additionals you have picked for individuals to make up their own fajitas. Take pleasure in!

CROWNING CHICKEN SALAD

THINGS NEEDED

75 g Natural yoghurt

Juice of 1/4 of a lemon

1 tea spoon. Coriander, sliced

1 teaspoon. Ground turmeric

1/2 teaspoon. Mild curry powder

100 g Cooked chicken breast, cut into bite-sized pieces

6 Walnut halves, carefully chopped

1 Medjool date, finely chopped

20 g Red onion, diced

1 Bird's eye chili

40 g Rocket, to dispense

ACTIONS

Mix the yogurt, lemon juice, coriander and spices together in a bowl. Consist of all the remaining things required and dish out on a bed of the rocket.

BUNLESS BEEF BURGERS WITH ALL THE TRIMMINGS

THINGS NEEDED

125 g Lean minced beef (5% fat).

15 g Red onion, finely chopped.

1 tea spoon. Parsley, finely sliced.

1 tea spoon. Extra virgin olive oil.

150 g Sweet potatoes.

1 tea spoon. Extra virgin olive oil.

1 tea spoon. Dried rosemary.

1 Garlic clove, unpeeled.

10 g Cheddar cheese, sliced or grated.

150 g Red onion, sliced into rings.

30 g Tomato, sliced.

10 g Rocket.

1 Gherkin (optional).

STEPS.

Heat the microwave oven to 220oC/gas 7.

Start by making the fries. Peel and cut the sweet potato into 1cm - thick chips. Toss them with the olive oil, increased mary and garlic clove. Place on a flat pan and roast for 30 minutes, until crispy and good.

For the hamburger, mix the onion and parsley with the minced beef. If you have pastry cutters, you might mould your hamburger with the largest pastry cutter in the set, otherwise, simply utilize your hands to make a nice even patty.

Heat a frying pan over a medium first heat, include the olive oil, then place the burger on one side of the pan and the onion rings on the other. Prepare the hamburger for 6 minutes on each side, guaranteeing it is prepared through. Fry the onion rings up until prepared to your taste.

When the burger is prepared, leading it with the cheese and red onion and place it in the hot microwave oven for a minute to melt the cheese. Remove and top with the rocket, gherkin and tomato. Dish out with the fries.

CHICKEN SKEWERS WITH SATAY SAUCE.

THINGS NEEDED.

150 g Chicken breast, cut into chunks.

1 tea spoon. Ground turmeric.

1/2 teaspoon. Extra virgin olive oil.

50 g Buckwheat.

30 g Kale, stalks eliminated and sliced.

30 g Celery, sliced.

4 Walnut halves, chopped, to garnish.

20 g Red onion, diced.

1 Garlic clove, sliced.

1 tea spoon. Bonus virgin olive oil.

1 tea spoon. Curry powder.

1 teaspoon. Ground turmeric.

50 ml Chicken stock.

150 ml Coconut milk.

1 table spoon. Walnut butter or peanut butter.

1 table spoon. Coriander, chopped.

ACTIONS.

Mix the chicken with the turmeric and olive oil and set aside to marinade-- 30 minutes to 1 hour would be best, however if you are short on time, just leave it for as long as you can.

Prepare the buckwheat according to the packet instructions, including the kale and celery for the last 5-- 7 minutes of the cooking time. Drain.

Very first heat the grill on a high setting.

For the sauce, gently fry the red onion and garlic in the olive oil for 2-- 3 minutes until soft. Consist of the spices and cook for a further minute. Include the stock and coconut milk and give the boil, then include the walnut butter and stir through. Decrease the very first heat and simmer the sauce for 8-- 10 minutes, or till creamy and abundant.

As the sauce is simmering, thread the chicken on to the skewers and place under the hot grill for 10 minutes, turning them after 5 minutes.

To dish out, stir the coriander through the sauce and pour it over the skewers, then scatter over the chopped walnuts.

SMOKED SALMON OMELETTE.

THINGS NEEDED.

2 Medium eggs.

100 g Smoked salmon, sliced.

1/2 tea spoon. Capers.

10 g Rocket, chopped.

1 tea spoon. Parsley, sliced.

1 tea spoon. Extra virgin olive oil.

STEPS.

Crack the eggs into a bowl and whisk well. Include the salmon, capers, rocket and parsley.

Heat the olive oil in a non-stick frying pan till hot but not smoking cigarettes. Include the egg mixture and, using a spatula or fish slice, move the mixture around the pan till it is even. Minimize the very first heat and let the omelette cook through. Move the spatula around the edges and roll up or fold the omelette in half to dispense.

DATE AND WALNUT PORRIDGE.

THINGS NEEDED.

200 ml Milk or dairy-free alternative.

1 Medjool date, chopped.

35 g Buckwheat flakes.

1 tea spoon. Walnut butter or 4 chopped walnut halves.

50 g Strawberries, hulled.

ACTIONS.

Place the milk and date in a pan, very first heat gently, then consist of the buckwheat flakes and cook until the porridge is your desired consistency.

Stir in the walnut butter or walnuts, leading with the strawberries and dish out.

BRAISED PUY LENTILS.

THINGS NEEDED.

8 Cherry tomatoes, cut in half.

2 tea spoon. Bonus virgin olive oil.

40 g Red onion, thinly sliced.

1 Garlic clove, carefully chopped.

40 g Celery, very finely sliced.

40 g Carrots, peeled and very finely sliced.

1 teaspoon. Paprika.

1 teaspoon. Thyme (dry or fresh).

75 g Puy lentils.

220 ml Vegetable stock.

50 g Kale, roughly sliced.

1 table spoon. Parsley, chopped.

20 g Rocket.

ACTIONS.

Very first heat your microwave oven to 120ºC/ gas 1/2.

Location the tomatoes into a small roasting tin and roast in the microwave for 35-- 45 minutes.

Heat a pan over a low-- medium very first heat. Include 1 teaspoon of the olive oil with the red onion, celery, garlic and carrot and fry for 1-- 2 minutes, up until softened. Stir in the paprika and thyme and cook for a more minute.

Wash the lentils in a fine-meshed sieve and include them to the pan in addition to the stock. Bring to the boil, then lower the very first heat and simmer carefully for 20 minutes with a cover on the pan. Offer the pan a stir every 7 minutes or so, including a little water if the level drops too much.

Include the kale and cook for a more 10 minutes. When the lentils are cooked, stir in the parsley and roasted tomatoes. Dish out with the rocket drizzled with the remaining teaspoon of olive oil.

PRAWN ARRABBIATA.

THINGS NEEDED.

Raw or prepared prawns (Ideally king prawns).

65 g Buckwheat pasta.

1 table spoon. Additional virgin olive oil.

40 g Red onion, carefully chopped.

1 Garlic clove, carefully chopped.

30 g Celery, carefully sliced.

1 Bird's eye chilli, carefully sliced.

1 tea spoon. Dried blended herbs.

1 tea spoon. Additional virgin olive oil.

2 table spoon. White red wine (optional).

400 g Tinned sliced tomatoes.

1 table spoon. Sliced parsley.

STEPS.

Fry the onion, garlic, chilli and celery and dried herbs in the oil over a medium-- low very first heat for 1-- 2 minutes. Turn the first heat up to medium, include the white wine and cook for 1 minute. Include the tomatoes and leave the sauce to simmer over a medium-low first heat for 20-- 30 minutes, till it has a nice abundant consistency. , if you feel the sauce is getting too thick just include a little water.

While the sauce is cooking bring a pan of water to the boil and cook the pasta according to the packet steps. When prepared to your liking, drain, toss with the olive oil and keep in the pan until needed.

If you are utilizing raw prawns include them to the sauce and cook for a more 3-- 4 minutes, until they have turned opaque and pink, include the parsley and dispense. Bring the sauce to the boil and dish out if you are utilizing prepared prawns include them with the parsley.

Include the cooked pasta to the sauce, mix thoroughly however gently and dish out.

TURMERIC BAKED SALMON.

THINGS NEEDED.

Skinned Salmon.

1 tea spoon. Extra virgin olive oil.

1 tea spoon. Ground turmeric.

1/4 Juice of a lemon.

1 tea spoon. Extra virgin olive oil.

40 g Red onion, carefully sliced.

60 g Tinned green lentils.

1 Garlic clove, carefully chopped.

1 Bire's eye chilli, finely sliced.

150 g Celery, cut into 2cm lengths.

1 tea spoon. Moderate curry powder.

130 g Tomato, cut into 8 wedges.

100 ml Chicken or veggie stock.

1 table spoon. Sliced parsley.

STEPS.

First heat the microwave to 200C/ gas mark 6.

Start with the spicy celery. Very first heat a fry pan over a medium-- low first heat, consist of the olive oil, then the onion, garlic, celery, ginger and chilli. Fry gently for 2-- 3 minutes or until softened however not coloured, then consist of the curry powder and cook for an additional minute.

Consist of the tomatoes then the stock and lentils and simmer carefully for 10 minutes. You might wish to increase or decrease the cooking time depending on how crunchy you like your celery.

Meanwhile, mix the turmeric, oil and lemon juice and rub over the salmon. Place on a baking tray and cook for 8-- 10 minutes.

To complete, stir the parsley through the celery and dish out with the salmon.

TUSCAN BEAN STEW.

Things needed:

1 table spoon additional virgin olive oil.

50g red onion, carefully sliced.

30g carrot, peeled and carefully chopped.

30g celery, cut and carefully chopped.

1 garlic clove, carefully sliced.

1/2 bird's eye chilli, finely sliced (optional).

1 tea spoon herbes de Provence.

200ml veggie stock.

1 x 400g tin chopped Italian tomatoes.

1 tea spoon tomato purée.

200g tinned combined beans.

50g kale, roughly sliced.

1 table spoon approximately chopped parsley.

40g buckwheat.

Guidelines:

Location the oil in a medium pan over a low--medium very first heat and gently fry the onion, carrot, celery, garlic, chilli, if using, and herbs, up until the onion is soft however not colored.

Include the stock, tomatoes and tomato purée and give the boil.

Consist of the beans and simmer for 30 minutes.

Include the kale and cook for another 5-- 10 minutes, until tender, then include the parsley.

On the other hand, cook the buckwheat according to the packet steps, drain and then dispense with the stew.

SIRTFOOD SNACKS

Exist any beneficial Sirtfood snacks? Snacking seems like a word loaded with negative connotations, conjuring pictures of sugar-loaded confectionary or salt-laden savoury products. The food market understands just too well our weak point for all things sweet, high and salted in fat, and conspires to ensure they are never ever far from eyeshot as we set about our everyday lives, an ever-present temptation.

Even if you're up for making a healthier choice, it's far from clear-cut, when treats marketed as 'all natural' or with 'no added sugar' can often be as high in sugars as their scrap food counterparts. The only distinction being that the sugars take place within the naturally sweet components they utilize instead of the act of sugarcoating itself. Have a look at the label and you'll quickly see that there can be spectacular quantities of sugar hidden away in so-called healthy treats in the form of honey, maple syrup, agave, dried fruits (but read on for more about dates later), and so on. The upshot is the very same-- it's still a high sugar snack, simply a whole lot more expensive.

As a result, snacks can typically wind up diminishing the dietary quality of the diet, when they might actually be a chance to favorably enhance it. So what should we be snacking on? Are they any Sirtfood snacks? There are a number of the leading 20 Sirtfoods that can be used as the basis for healthy Sirtfood snacks.

Nuts have to be the stereotypical healthy junk food, packed with 'good' unsaturated fats, plant protein, fiber, and a wealth of vitamins, polyphenols, and minerals. With credentials like that it's no surprise that frequently eating nuts slashes the risk of cardiovascular disease. And in complete contrast to other high fat treats, frequently eating nuts is linked to having a slimmer waistline, likely due to their powerful satiating result. Walnuts, in specific are an effective sirtuin-activating food and a nice Sirtfood treat. Most importantly nuts are handbag and workplace desk friendly.

Next in the snacking stakes, and the ideal partner to nuts, is dark chocolate (preferably with an 80-85% cocoa material). Integrate a few squares of dark chocolate with a little handful of nuts and you have just about the most cardio-protective snack going.

As part of the Sirtfood Diet these Dark Chocolate Bites are a company household preferred as one of the nicest Sirtfood treats. It integrates a host of health promoting polyphenols into an indulgent treat. Whilst Medjool dates are naturally very high in sugar (an incredible 66%!), eaten in moderation they really have no obvious blood glucose raising impacts and are in fact connected to having less diabetes and cardiovascular disease, thanks to their exceptional polyphenol material. This makes them among the healthiest choices for creating a sweet reward.

Here are nine easy Sirtfood snacks you can reach for when you need a SIRT top-up.

1 Green tea

1 cup (200ml) • 1 of your SIRT 5 a day • 0 calories

Never, ever, underestimate the healthy SIRT boost that a cup of green tea can give you. Have as many cups as you can per day – we recommend at least two cups. Not only that, the SIRTs in green tea are cumulative so you can get up to four portions of SIRTs daily if you have four cups of green tea or more.

2 Red grapes

10 grapes • 1 of your SIRT 5 a day • 30 calories

Another of the very easy Sirtfood snacks and a low-calorie way to get one of your SIRT portions. Keep a punnet or two in the fridge and have a handful at breakfast or lunch or even both!

3 Apples

1 apple • 1 of your SIRT 5 a day • 47 calories

An apple a day really does keep the doctor away. Reach for an apple as one of your after-lunch easy Sirtfood snacks. It will help keep sugar cravings at bay too.

4 Cocoa

2 tsp/10g cocoa • 1 of your SIRT 5 a day • 33 calories

Try making a chocolate shot with 2 tsp cocoa. 1 tsp sugar and 30ml milk. Mix the cocoa and sugar with a little boiling water from the kettle to make a smooth paste. Stir in the milk. An (almost) instant chocolate hit with only 68 calories.

5 Olives

6 large black or green olives • 1 of your SIRT 5 a day • 75 calories

A versatile and easy Sirtfood snack in the afternoon or a pre-dinner treat. Serve at room temperature to get a fuller flavor.

6 Blackberries

15 blackberries • 1 of your SIRT 5 a day • 32 calories

Another of the easy Sirtfood snacks to keep in your fridge. Also great as a frozen treat.

7 Dark chocolate 85%

6 squares/20g chocolate • 1 of your SIRT 5 a day • 125 calories

Get your chocolate hit here! If you prefer 70% dark chocolate, you'll need 9 squares/30g. which will be 180 calories.

8 Pomegranate seeds

50g/half a small pack • 1 of your SIRT 5 a day • 50 calories

Easy to obtain while on the go, pomegranate seeds pack a large SIRT punch and you only need half a 100g pack to get one of your SIRT portions.

9 Blueberries

25 blueberries (80g) • 1 of your sirt 5 a day • 36 cals

One large handful of blueberries can also be one of your easy Sirtfood snacks

ARE SIRTFOODS THE NEW SUPERFOODS?

There's no denying that sirtfoods benefit you. They are frequently high in nutrients and complete healthy plant compounds.

Moreover, research studies have associated many of the foods recommended on the Sirtfood Diet with health advantages.

For example, consuming moderate amounts of dark chocolate with high cocoa content might decrease the danger of cardiovascular disease and assistance fight inflammation.

Consuming green tea might decrease the risk of stroke and diabetes and help lower high blood pressure.

And turmeric has anti-inflammatory properties that have advantageous impacts on the body in general and may even secure against chronic, inflammation-related illness).

The bulk of sirtfoods have demonstrated health benefits in people.

Nevertheless, proof of the health advantages of increasing sirtuin protein levels is preliminary. Research in animals and cell lines has revealed exciting results.

For instance, researchers have found that increased levels of certain sirtuin proteins cause longer lifespan in yeast, mice, and worms.

And throughout fasting or calorie limitation, sirtuin proteins inform the body to burn more fat for energy and improve insulin level of sensitivity. One study in mice discovered that increased sirtuin levels resulted in weight loss.

Some evidence recommends that sirtuins may likewise play a role in minimizing swelling, hindering the advancement of growths, and slowing the development of cardiovascular disease and Alzheimer's.

While research studies in mice and human cell lines have revealed favorable results, there have been no human studies examining the effects of increasing sirtuin levels.

Whether increasing sirtuin protein levels in the body will lead to longer life-span or a lower danger of cancer in humans is unknown.

A research study is currently underway to develop substances efficient at increasing sirtuin levels in the body. By doing this, human research studies can begin to take a look at the effects of sirtuins on human health

Until then, it's not possible to identify the results of increased sirtuin levels.

Sirtfoods are generally healthy foods.

Extremely little is understood about how these foods affect sirtuin levels and human health.

IS IT HEALTHY AND SUSTAINABLE?

Sirtfoods are nearly all healthy options and may even lead to some health benefits due to their anti-inflammatory or antioxidant residential or commercial properties.

Yet consuming simply a handful of particularly healthy foods can not satisfy all of your body's dietary needs.

The Sirtfood Diet is needlessly restrictive and uses no clear, special health benefits over any other kind of diet.

Eating only 1,000 calories is normally not suggested without the supervision of a physician. Even consuming 1,500 calories per day is exceedingly limiting for many individuals.

The diet plan also needs draining to 3 green juices per days. Although juices can be a good source of minerals and vitamins, they are likewise a source of sugar and consist of nearly none of the healthy fiber that whole fruits and veggies do

What's more, sipping on juice throughout the whole day is a bad concept for both your blood sugar and your teeth.

Not to point out, because the diet plan is so minimal in calories and food choice, it is more than most likely lacking in protein, vitamins, and minerals, specifically during the first stage.

Due to the low-calorie levels and limiting food options, this diet plan may be challenging to adhere to for the whole three weeks.

Add that to the high initial expenses of needing to buy a juicer, the book, and specific uncommon and costly components, in addition to the time expenses of preparing specific meals and juices, and this diet plan ends up being unfeasible and unsustainable for many individuals.

The Sirtfood Diet promotes healthy foods but is limiting in calories and food choices. It likewise involves drinking great deals of juice, which isn't a healthy suggestion.

SAFETY AND SIDE EFFECTS

Although the first phase of the Sirtfood Diet is very low in calories and nutritionally incomplete, there are no genuine safety issues for the average, healthy adult thinking about the diet plan's brief duration.

Yet for somebody with diabetes, calorie limitation and drinking primarily juice for the very first couple of days of the diet might cause hazardous modifications in blood glucose levels.

Even a healthy individual may experience some side results-- generally hunger.

Eating just 1,000-- 1,500 calories per day will leave practically anybody sensation starving, particularly if much of what you're taking in is juice, which is low in fiber, a nutrient that helps keep you feeling complete.

Throughout phase one, you might experience opposite effects such as fatigue, irritability, and lightheadedness due to the calorie limitation.

For the otherwise healthy adult, major health consequences are unlikely if the diet plan is followed for just three weeks.

The Sirtfood Diet is low in calories and phase one is not nutritionally well balanced. It may leave you hungry, however, it's not harmful to the average healthy grownup.

CONCLUSION

Time and time once again, I've explained to you guys the problem with the majority of diets: restrictive consuming. When it pertains to constraint, our rebel impulses desire to stick it to the guy and binge like crazy. I'm quite sure you'll also become that good friend that nobody desires to go out with because of your brand-new hangry character. For realsies, there have not been sufficient constant research studies that say calorie limitation is the way to go. Sure, you'll lose some sweet poundage briefly however you'll also fulfill some undesirable outcomes and ultimately restore the weight. Research studies looking at caloric constraint discovered that in time limitation results in loss of muscle mass (which completely counters what the sirtfood diet plan claims it can do), muscle strength and loss of bone, anemia, depression, and irritation.

The most significant claim this diet boasts about is that these sirtuin proteins will increase our body's ability to burn fat, promote muscle repair work, growth and upkeep and as pointed out earlier- quick weight-loss. Right?! (insert enormous eye roll) because rapid weight loss is always safe. Other non-weight associated advantages consist of: improving memory, managing blood sugar level levels, and protecting you from cancers and persistent illness.

The Sirtfood diet stresses consuming foods that might engage with a household of proteins known as sirtuin proteins (now the name of the diet plan is starting to make sense). Since of the role they play in the metabolic process, some professionals are calling sirtuins "slim genes" for their prospective function in weight loss.

Sirtfoods promote sirtuin genes, which are stated to influence the body's capability to burn fat and boost the metabolic system.

The Sirtfood diet plan is based upon 2 stages;

Phase one is an intensive seven-day program developed to kick-start your intense weight reduction.

Then stage 2 has to do with upping the amount of Sirtfood-rich fruit and vegetables in your everyday meals to preserve weight-loss.

Unlike numerous other short-term yo-yo diets, the Sirtfood plan includes meals and guidance on how to keep off the weight you lose in the very first week by continuing to incorporate Sirtfoods as part of a well balanced and healthy diet plan.

DISCLAIMER

This book is not intended as a substitute for the medical advice of physicians. The reader should regularly consult a physician in matters relating to his/her health and particularly concerning any symptoms that may require diagnosis or medical attention.

(diet, sirtfood)

ABOUT THE AUTHOR

MY NAME IS

Sam Gareth

I really love educating people on how to stay
healthy and live the life of their dreams.

Do Not Go Yet; One Last Thing To Do

If you enjoyed this book or found it useful, I'd be very grateful if you'd post a short review on Amazon. Your support does make a difference, and I read all the reviews personally so I can get your feedback and make this book even better.

Thanks again for your support!

Printed in Germany
by Amazon Distribution
GmbH, Leipzig

18014677R00145